PROGRESS IN CLINICAL AND BIOLOGICAL RESEARCH

RECENT TITLES

See pages following the index for previous titles in this series.

ONCOGENES AND RETROVIRUSES

Evaluation of Basic Findings and Clinical Potential

ONCOGENES AND RETROVIRUSES

Evaluation of Basic Findings and Clinical Potential

**Proceedings of a Workshop held at
Roswell Park Memorial Institute
Buffalo, New York, September 2–3, 1982**

Editors

TIMOTHY E. O'CONNOR
Roswell Park Memorial Institute
Buffalo, New York

FRANK J. RAUSCHER, JR.
American Cancer Society
New York, New York

ALAN R. LISS, INC. • NEW YORK

Address all Inquiries to the Publisher
Alan R. Liss, Inc., 150 Fifth Avenue, New York, NY 10011

Copyright © 1983 Alan R. Liss, Inc.
Printed in the United States of America.

Library of Congress Cataloging in Publication Data

Main entry under title:

Oncogenes and retroviruses.
  (Progress in clinical and biological research; v. 119)
  Includes bibliographies and index.
  1. Viral carcinogenesis--Genetic aspects--Congresses.
2. Oncogenes--Congresses. 3. Viruses, RNA--Congresses.
I. O'Connor, Timothy E.   II. Rauscher, Frank J.
III. Roswell Park Memorial Institute.   IV. Title:
Retroviruses.   V. Series.   [DNLM: 1. Oncogenes--Congresses.
2. Retroviridae--Congresses. W1 PR668E v.119 / QW 166
058 1982]
RC268.57.048   1983   616.99'4071   83-694
ISBN 0-8451-0119-6

Contents

Contributors

Stuart A. Aaronson [207]
Laboratory of Cellular and Molecular Biology, National Cancer Institute, Bethesda, Maryland 20205

Garth R. Anderson [185]
Department of Cell and Tumor Biology, Roswell Park Memorial Institute, Buffalo, New York 14263

David Baltimore [57]
Whitehead Institute for Biomedical Research, Massachusetts Institute of Technology, Cambridge, Massachusetts 02139

D.G. Blair [79]
Laboratory of Molecular Oncology, Frederick Cancer Research Facility, Frederick, Maryland 21701

Alexander Bloch [264]
Department of Experimental Therapeutics, Grace Cancer Drug Center, Roswell Park Memorial Institute, Buffalo, New York 14263

Dani Paul Bolognesi [257]
Department of Surgery, Duke University Medical Center, Durham, North Carolina 27710

Joan S. Brugge [135]
Department of Microbiology, State University of New York, Stony Brook, New York 11794

John J. Burns [266]
Research Division, Hoffman-La Roche Inc., Nutley, New Jersey 07110

Peter Centner [149]
Paul-Ehrlich-Institut, D-6000 Frankfurt, Federal Republic of Germany

R.S.K. Chaganti [119]
Memorial Sloan-Kettering Cancer Center, New York, New York 10021

J.W. Chamberlain [173]
Department of Biochemistry, McGill University, Montreal, Quebec, Canada H3G 1Y6

I.S.Y. Chen [43]
Division of Hematology/Oncology, UCLA School of Medicine, Los Angeles, California 90024

J.M. Coffin [37]
Department of Molecular Biology and Microbiology, Tufts University School of Medicine, Boston, Massachusetts 02111

The boldface number in brackets following a contributor's name is the opening page number of that contributors paper.

x / Contributors

C.S. Cooper [79]
Laboratory of Molecular Oncology, National Cancer Institute, Bethesda,
Maryland 20205

B. Cullen [105]
Hoffmann-La Roche Inc., Nutley, New Jersey 07110

Diane Darrow [135]
Department of Microbiology, State University of New York, Stony Brook,
New York 11794

Deborah DeFeo [67]
Department of Virus and Cell Research, Merck Sharpe and Dohme Research
Laboratories, West Point, Pennsylvania 19486

Claire Y. Dunn [207]
Laboratory of Cellular and Molecular Biology, National Cancer Institute,
Bethesda, Maryland 20205

L.A. Eader [79]
NIH Intramural Research Support Program, NCI-Frederick Cancer Research
Facility, Frederick, Maryland 21701

Erich Eigenbrodt [149]
Institut für Biochemie und Endokrinologie, D-6300 Giessen,
Federal Republic of Germany

Ronald W. Ellis [67]
Department of Virus and Cell Research, Merck Sharpe and Dohme Research
Laboratories, West Point, Pennsylvania 19486

Nelson W. Ellmore [207]
Laboratory of Cellular and Molecular Biology, National Cancer Institute,
Bethesda, Maryland 20205

Myron Essex [257]
Department of Microbiology, Harvard School of Public Health, Boston,
Massachusetts 02115

Alessandra Eva [207]
Laboratory of Cellular and Molecular Biology, National Cancer Institute,
Bethesda, Maryland 20205

Mary Jo Evans [185]
Roswell Park Memorial Institute, Buffalo, New York 14263

Peter J. Fischinger [256]
National Cancer Institute, National Institutes of Health, Bethesda,
Maryland 20205

Robert R. Friis [149]
Institut für Virologie, FB Humanmedizin, D-6300 Giessen,
Federal Republic of Germany

George J. Galasso [265]
Microbiology and Infectious Diseases Program, National Institute of Allergy
and Infectious Diseases, Bethesda, Maryland 20205

Robert C. Gallo [223]
Laboratory of Tumor Cell Biology, National Cancer Institute, Bethesda,
Maryland 20205

Jordan U. Gutterman [267]
Department of Developmental Therapeutics, University of Texas Cancer Center, Houston, Texas 77030

William S. Hayward [119]
Laboratory of Genetics and Oncology, Sloan-Kettering Institute for Cancer Research, New York, New York 10021

Alan N. Houghton [199]
Memorial Sloan-Kettering Cancer Center, New York, New York 10021

L. Jensen [37]
Worcester Foundation for Experimental Biology, Shrewsbury, Massachusetts 01545

S.C. Jhanwar [119]
Memorial Sloan-Kettering Cancer Center, New York, New York 10021

G. Ju [105]
Hoffmann-La Roche Inc., Nutley, New Jersey 07110

Henry S. Kaplan [254]
Department of Radiology, Stanford University Medical Center, Stanford, California 94305

Werner H. Kirsten [255]
Department of Pathology, University of Chicago, Chicago, Illinois 60637

T. Lam [173]
The Ontario Cancer Institute, Toronto, Ontario, Canada M4X 1K9

Arnold J. Levine [159]
Department of Microbiology, State University of New York, Stony Brook, New York 11794

Arthur D. Levinson [259]
Department of Molecular Biology, Genentech, Inc., South San Francisco, California 94080

Leah A. Lipsich [135]
Department of Microbiology, State University of New York, Stony Brook, New York 11794

R. Malavarca [105]
Roche Institute of Molecular Biology, Nutley, New Jersey 07110

Kenneth F. Manly [185]
Roswell Park Memorial Institute, Buffalo, New York 14263

Enrico Mihich [262]
Department of Experimental Therapeutics, Grace Cancer Drug Center, Roswell Park Memorial Institute, Buffalo, New York 14263

Arnold I. Mittelman [264]
Department of Surgical Oncology, Roswell Park Memorial Institute, Buffalo, New York 14263

Isao Miyoshi [243]
Department of Medicine, Kochi Medical School, Kochi 781-51, Japan

Gerald P. Murphy [xvii]
Director, Roswell Park Memorial Institute, Buffalo, New York 14263

B.G. Neel [119]
Memorial Sloan-Kettering Cancer Center, New York, New York 10021

Timothy E. O'Connor [xix, 1]
Associate Director for Scientific Affairs, Roswell Park Memorial Institute,
Buffalo, New York 14263

Yuji Ohtsuki [243]
Kochi Medical School, Kochi 781-51, Japan

M.K. Oskarsson [79]
Laboratory of Molecular Oncology, National Cancer Institute, Bethesda,
Maryland 20205

Howard Ozer [260]
Department of Medical Oncology, Roswell Park Memorial Institute, Buffalo,
New York 14263

Alex Papageorge [67]
Department of Virus and Cell Research, Merck Sharpe and Dohme Research
Laboratories, West Point, Pennsylvania 19486

James K. Petell [185]
Roswell Park Memorial Institute, Buffalo, New York 14263

Victoria R. Polonis [185]
Roswell Park Memorial Institute, Buffalo, New York 14263

Harvey D. Preisler [263]
Department of Medical Oncology, Roswell Park Memorial Institute, Buffalo,
New York 14263

G.B. Price [173]
Cancer Centre, McGill University, Montreal, Quebec, Canada H3G 1Y6

Ron Prywes [57]
Whitehead Institute for Biomedical Research, Massachusetts Institute of
Technology, Cambridge, Massachusetts 02139

Frank J. Rauscher, Jr. [xix, 253]
American Cancer Society, Inc., New York, New York 10017

Nancy Reich [159]
Department of Microbiology, State University of New York, Stony Brook,
New York 11794

H.L. Robinson [37]
Cell Biology Group, Worcester Foundation for Experimental Biology,
Shrewsbury, Massachusetts 01545

Helga Rübsamen [149]
Department of Virology, Paul-Ehrlich-Institut, D-6000 Frankfurt,
Federal Republic of Germany

Raul Saavedra [185]
Roswell Park Memorial Institute, Buffalo, New York 14263

Ruth Sager [259]
Division of Cancer Genetics, Sidney Farber Cancer Institute, Boston,
Massachusetts 02115

Alan Y. Sakaguchi [93]
Department of Human Genetics, Roswell Park Memorial Institute, Buffalo,
New York 14263

P. Schatz [37]
Massachusetts Institute of Technology, Cambridge, Massachusetts 02139

Edward M. Scolnick [67]
Department of Virus and Cell Research, Merck, Sharpe and Dohme Research Laboratories, West Point, Pennsylvania 19486

P.R. Shank [37]
Brown University, Providence, Rhode Island 02912

C.-K. Shih [119]
Memorial Sloan-Kettering Cancer Center, New York, New York 10021

Yukimasa Shiraishi [243]
Kochi Medical School, Kochi 781-51, Japan

Thomas B. Shows [261]
Department of Human Genetics, Roswell Park Memorial Institute, Buffalo, New York 14263

A.M. Skalka [105]
Roche Institute of Molecular Biology, Nutley, New Jersey 07110

C.P. Stanners [173]
Department of Biochemistry, McGill University, Montreal, Quebec, Canada H3G 1Y6

Hirokuni Taguchi [243]
Kochi Medical School, Kochi 781-51, Japan

H.M. Temin [43]
McArdle Laboratory for Cancer Research, University of Wisconsin, Madison, Wisconsin 53706

Rees Thomas [159]
Department of Microbiology, State University of New York, Stony Brook, New York 11794

P.N. Tsichlis [37,105]
Laboratory of Tumor Virus Genetics, National Cancer Institute, Bethesda, Maryland 20205

G.F. Vande Woude [79]
Laboratory for Molecular Oncology, National Cancer Institute, Bethesda, Maryland 20205

Harold E. Varmus [23]
Department of Microbiology and Immunology, University of California, San Francisco, California 94143

Jean Yin Jen Wang [57]
Whitehead Institute for Biomedical Research, Massachusetts Institute of Technology, Cambridge, Massachusetts 02139

K.C. Wilhelmsen [43]
McArdle Laboratory for Cancer Research, University of Wisconsin, Madison, Wisconsin 53706

Flossie Wong-Staal [223]
Laboratory of Tumor Cell Biology, National Cancer Institute, Bethesda, Maryland 20205

Wes Yonemoto [135]
Department of Microbiology, State University of New York, Stony Brook, New York 11794

Distinguished Visitors

Joel Bennett
  Pharmaceutical Advisory Board
Roland Berger
  St. Louis Hospital, Paris
Mrs. William McC. Blair
  Lasker Foundation
Ken Blank
  University of Pennsylvania Medical
  School
Theodore T. Bronk
  Mount St. Mary's Hospital
Temesa Chan-Castillo
  Veterans Administration Hospital
Fernando De Noronha
  Cornell University
Irene M. Evans
  University of Rochester
Alice Fordyce
  Lasker Foundation
James Fordyce
  Lasker Foundation
Albert J. Frey
  Sandoz, Inc.
L. Patrick Gage
  Hoffmann-La Roche, Inc.
Cynthia M. Greaton
  Columbia University
Robert Greene
  Niagara University
Gary Hahn
  Erie County Medical Center
Gavin Hildick-Smith
  Johnson & Johnson

Leo Kim
  Shell Oil Company
William J. Kokolus
  State University of New York,
  Buffalo
Mary Lasker
  Lasker Foundation
Rene Le Strange
  Sloan-Kettering
Harold Lehman
  Veterans Administration Hospital
Leorosa Lehman
  Veterans Administration Hospital
Leon Lewandowski
  Laboratory Medicine Institute
Max Link
  Sandoz, Inc.
Richard Love
  Shell Oil Company
Sharon McAiliffe
  New York Times Magazine
Fernandino Merino
  Venezuela Cancer Center
Ricardo Mesa-Tejada
  Columbia University
Richard Montagna
  Cellular Products
Donna Murasko
  Medical College of Pennsylvania
Tsuneya Ohno
  Columbia University
Allen Oliff
  Sloan Kettering

William Pinkel
American Cancer Society, NYS Division
Bernard Poiesz
Upstate Medical Center
Harold Schmeck
New York Times
Edith Sproul
Pathology Consultant, Roswell Park Memorial Institute
Gerald Sufrin
State University of New York, Buffalo

Robert Sutherland
University of Rochester
Robert Ting
Biosystems
Herman Van de Rerghe
University of Leuben, Brussels
Kristin White
Author, New York City
William Zapisek
Canisus College

Welcome and Introduction

Gerald P. Murphy, MD, DSc
Institute Director
Roswell Park Memorial Institute

"I welcome all the participants in this workshop to this important scientific meeting on the 'Onc-Sarc Gene'. I can think of no more exciting field than this particular area at this moment. The very fact that members of over 35 laboratories from all over the world were able to gather within a few weeks notice, emphasizes both the importance and timeliness of this particular topic and, as well, the interest of other scientists of diverse backgrounds in addressing it. I wish to compliment both Dr. Rauscher and Dr. O'Connor who will, as co-chairmen of the Workshop and subsequent Proceedings, see to it that it is rapidly produced or 'replicated' if you will. I also think it is most fitting to acknowledge the timely support of the American Cancer Society, which has made it possible for Roswell Park Memorial Institute to host this important conference at this time. We look forward to a most successful conclusion and, to be sure, even more rapid subsequent developments."

Foreword

Over the past seven years research in cell biology and virology has led to unexpected and exciting insights into the role of genes in cell regulation and in production of neoplasia. Among the new findings was the discovery that the RNA-containing retroviruses, which can rapidly transform cells in culture, contain genes (v-onc genes) which are closely related to genes that occur in all vertebrate species (c-onc genes). Other interesting findings include the delineation of the terminal regions of integrated retroviral DNA (LTRs) as regions which contain several of the control elements for gene expression. From these findings has arisen an active study of the interaction of the LTR segments and the cellular and viral onc genes and the role of these interactions in neoplasia. This activity in turn has led to the examination, as yet incomplete, of the protein products which are encoded by the cellular and viral onc genes. Already these findings have given a preliminary picture of some of the molecular lesions involved in animal and human neoplasia. The present Workshop was convened to place these various developments in perspective and in particular to evaluate their utility for human benefit. We trust that the present volume will serve as a record of a very exciting Workshop in which significant advances in our understanding of cancer were presented. It is our hope that this new information will provide a stimulus to the further development of improved procedures for the diagnosis and treatment of cancer.

Timothy E. O'Connor
Frank J. Rauscher, Jr.

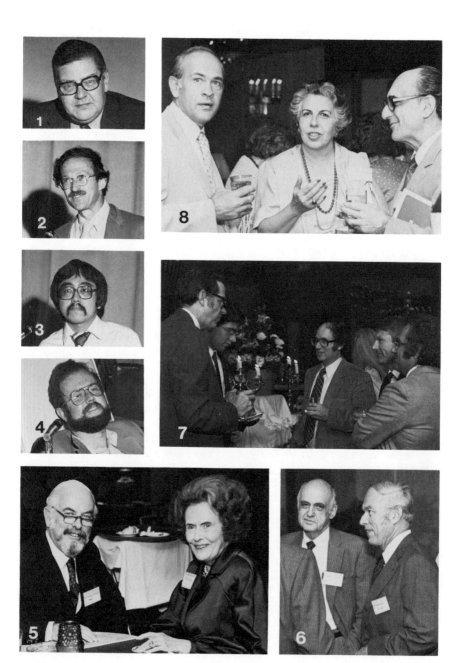

1. F. Rauscher; 2. H. Varmus; 3. A. Sakaguchi; 4. G. Anderson; 5. T. O'Connor, M. Lasker; 6. M. Hilleman, H. Schmeck; 7. E. Henderson, F. Rauscher III, T. Beerman, J. Bertram, Y. Rustum; 8. D. Bolognesi, Mrs. and Dr. E. Mihich.

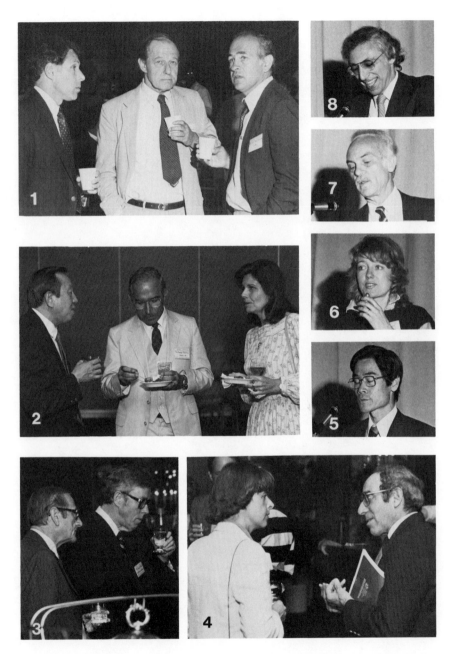

1. S. Aaronson, W. Kirsten, D. Bolognesi; 2. R. Ting, G. Galasso, K. White; 3. G. Hildick-Smith, J. Burns; 4. B. Henderson, A. Bloch; 5. I. Miyoshi; 6. H. Rübsamen; 7. R. Hutter; 8. R. Gallo.

Oncogenes and Retroviruses: Evaluation of Basic Findings and Clinical Potential, pages 1–19

MOLECULAR LESIONS ASSOCIATED WITH NEOPLASIA: AN INTRODUC-
TION TO PROVIRUSES, RETROVIRUSES, LTR'S AND ONC GENES

Timothy E. O'Connor, Ph.D.

Associate Institute Director for Scientific
Affairs, Roswell Park Memorial Institute, 666
Elm Street, Buffalo, N.Y. 14263

Six years have now elapsed since the first definitive
demonstration by Stahelin, Varmus, Bishop and Vogt that
cells of the normal uninfected chicken, quail and other
avian species contain DNA with nucleotide sequences
(c-onc) that are homologous to the transforming gene
(v-onc) of avian sarcoma virus. This finding of the
existence of a cellular onc gene and its close relatedness
to a viral onc gene (v-onc) was soon followed by the
demonstration that cells of all vertebrates contain copies
of DNA that are closely homologous to the transforming
genes of each of the acutely transforming retroviruses.
These findings came at a time when a wealth of information
had accumulated on the biology of retroviruses in a range
of animal species and when new techniques (e.g.
recombinant DNA, rapid DNA sequencing, and monoclonal
antibody) had vastly enriched the armentarium of the
researcher. The result has been an explosion in
information. The purpose of this meeting is to evaluate
this information and, in particular, with respect to its
potential for the understanding, prevention and treatment
of human cancer. My task is to provide an overview of
some of these developments. My hope is that this brief
review will provide the non-specialist with a broad
perspective on the developments and some of the
terminologies and techniques employed. For the specialist
it may provide an opportunity for distinguishing the wood
from the trees, or at least, a period for quiet
transcendental meditation.

As illustrated in Figure 1, modern biology permits us

to view the cell as a computer-controlled protein factory. In this factory the various genes, A, B, C, etc.

Cell As Computer-Controlled Protein Factory

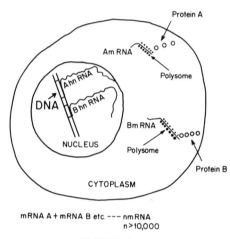

mRNA A + mRNA B etc. --- nmRNA
n > 10,000

FIGURE 1

are encoded in the double stranded DNA of the nucleus and are then transcribed individually into heterogeneous RNA. This hnRNA is then processed and transported to the cytoplasm where it is translated on polysomes to yield the respective proteins A, B, C, D, etc. While this scheme is straightforward, the range of products is large. Thus, examinations of proteins yielded by the cells of specific tissues show more than 5,000 proteins per cell.
Similarly, analysis of the heterogeneity of the mRNA in the cells reveals an excess of 10,000 different species in typical cells of any tissue. Nevertheless, this mRNA on the basis of hybridization experiments to the DNA of the nucleus has been shown to comprise only approximately 3% of the total DNA in the nucleus. Furthermore, cells from different tissues show overlap and differences in their mRNA content (Davidson, 1976). Thus a central question in modern biology is the nature of the controls which determine which particular genes are to be transcribed and at what level, and thus provide the particular phenotype of the cell.

We must also note that a vertebrate organism is not static but develops from the fertilized ovum through intermediate stages to the final mature organism. Experiments in developmental biology have indicated that from the stage of the fertilized ovum to the blastocyst all the inner cells retain total developmental capacity and can thus ultimately develop into any mature tissue in the mature organism. At later stages in the embryonic development specific tissues develop. At this stage the cells are committed and can develop only along lineages which ultimately lead to the terminally differentiated cell. One view of neoplasia is that the neoplastic cell arises through an error in the terminal differentiation process during normal tissue renewal (Pierce, B., 1972). Among the topics that will be considered in this Workshop will be the potential role of onc genes and their products in controlling the cellular phenotype and the potential use of this knowledge in diagnosis and treatment of cancer.

The biology of onc genes must be viewed in the context of the biology of retroviruses which is summarized in Figure 2. Retroviruses are membrane-enclosed viruses which bud from the cell membrane of infected cells and which do not generally kill the cells which they infect. The viral genome consists of two identical strands of RNA, one of which is shown in Figure 2, and which are held

Retrovirus Biology

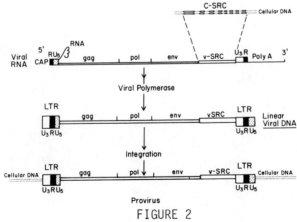

FIGURE 2

together by tRNA molecules. The viral RNA of all retroviruses contain nucleotide sequences which are ultimately expressed as internal virion proteins (gag region), external virus-membrane glycopeptide (env), and a virus-associated polymerase (pol). Antisera to these proteins generally provide the virologist with a rapid and definitive characterization of the species of origin and type of a particular virus isolate. Retroviruses are however unique among animal viruses in four respects: (a) Their unique mode of replication through an intermediate proviral DNA and integration into the host-cell DNA; (b) The capacity of the integrated provirus to be transmitted through somatic or germ cells as a cellular gene; (c) The presence of repeat nucleotide sequences at both ends of the viral RNA and in integrated proviral DNA. These terminal LTR sequences in the proviral DNA contain regulatory signals for initiation of transcription and for placing a poly A sequence on the hnRNA transcript; (d) and the capacity of non-acute retroviruses to recombine with modified cellular regulatory genes (c-oncs) to provide acutely transforming viruses which then contain the modified v-onc gene.

Since the "molecular gymnastics" of retrovirus replication have recently been reviewed (Varmus, 1982) only the highlights will receive comment here. The replication of the viral RNA into double stranded DNA is mediated by the viral polymerase ("reverse transcriptase"). The ensuing linear or circular DNA is then inserted at random, but in a constant orientation, into the host cell genome. The viral RNA contains at both the 5' and 3' termini short Direct Repeats (R) of nucleotide sequences and also adjacent regions (U5 and U3 respectively) which each contain Inverted Repeats of nucleotide sequences. Note that in the course of replication a U3 sequence is added at the 5' end of the proviral DNA and a U5 sequence is added at the 3' end of the proviral DNA. Thus the proviral DNA consists of a number of gene-coding sequences of DNA that are flanked by identical termini – the LTR regions – which do not encode for proteins and which contain U3:R:U5 sequences in a 5'-3' orientation. It may also be noted that the virologist in his experimentation can obtain radioactively labeled DNA transcripts that are respectively homologous to the LTR, whole virus, or whole virus minus the v-onc regions. Such probes can be used to detect the intact or partial proviral DNA in cells through hybridization experiments. Furthermore, these DNA transcripts can be

cut at specific restriction enzyme sites and cloned into
bacterial hosts via appropriate virus or plasmid vectors.

The features described above are common to all
retroviruses. Retroviruses which can rapidly transform
appropriate cells to the malignant phenotype and rapidly
induce tumors on infection – the acutely-transforming
viruses – also contain an RNA segment (v-onc) which codes
for the cellular transformation. Construction of a c-DNA
probe complementary to this region of the RNA of the
acutely-transforming Rous chicken sarcoma virus (V-src)
facilitated the demonstration of the presence of a
homologous but distinct gene (c-sarc) in the cells of all
vertebrates that were tested (Stehelin et al.). The
melting characteristics of the v-src/c-sarc DNA hybrids
indicated strong conservation of these sequences in
animals over a wide time-frame of evolution. Cellular DNA
sequences homologous to the transforming genes of other
acute transformation viruses were rapidly delineated.
Some, like the c-src shown in Figure 3, contained intron
regions of DNA interspersed between the coding DNA
sequences. Others (e.g. c-mos) do not show the presence
of introns. The modest changes in nucleotide sequence and
in the structure of the proteins encoded by the respective
c-onc and v-onc genes is receiving close scrutiny. The
isolation of only fourteen v-onc genes to date despite the
diligence of the virologists, and the frequent recovery of
the same v-onc genes in several independent isolations of
retroviruses, suggests that the number of corresponding
c-onc genes is relatively small. The c-onc genes
therefore appear to provide very useful markers amid the
great diversity of the genome-content of vertebrate
organisms. A richer appreciation of the biological
significance of these genes may emerge from further
consideration of the roles of cellular provirus; the
properties of LTR DNA segments; infectious retrovirus and
its capacity to generate recombinant viruses; and the
specific properties of the protein products of the c-onc
and v-onc genes.

Once the provirus is integrated into the DNA of the
cell, its subsequent behavior is similar to that of other
cellular genes. Infection of the germ cells of an animal
can ultimately result in progeny in which every cell will
contain a copy of the provirus. Inheritance of such
proviruses follows Mendelian pattern. Evidence exists

that the env gene in the provirus may ultimately code for
a protein present as a glycopeptide in the membranes of
certain cells which behaves as an alloantigen and which
may determine the outcome of differentiation. A typical
example of this is the presence of the GIX antigen as
glycopeptide in the membranes of thymus cells of certain
mouse strains and which is encoded by the env gene of the
Gross leukemia virus and which is expressed at high levels
in Gross mouse and rat leukemias (Stockert et al., 1971).
It is important to note that the outcome of infection with
a retrovirus critically depends upon the stage in
embryonic development at which the infection occurs
(Jahner et al., 1982). Thus infection of the zygote or
preimplantation embryo results in integration of the
provirus but no infectious virus is produced. It has been
shown that the integrated virus is heavily methylated.
Normal animals can result from such infections but the
provirus remains silent and highly methylated. In
contrast, when mouse embryo is infected at a later stage,
at approximately day 8 of embryogenesis, the integrated
provirus is not methylated, infectious virus is produced
and rapidly spreads from cell to cell and infects all
cells of the organism. In contrast, when neonatal animals
are infected the provirus is predominantly integrated into
cells of particular lineages and may ultimately produce
neoplasia. Integrated proviruses obviously provide highly
attractive candidates for the study of gene regulation.
In this connection it has been noted that activation of
the mouse mammary tumor virus involves demethylation
(Breznik and Cohen, 1982). Likewise, a silent provirus of
the chicken, ev-1 can be activated by exposure to the drug
5-azacytidine whereupon hypomethylation ensues.
Simultaneously a DNAse I sensitive site is generated in
the LTR region of the provirus (Groudine et al., 1981).

Since the LTR DNA segments play such a role in the
biology of retroviruses they merit a closer scrutiny. As
mentioned earlier, viral replication involves the
generation of an LTR region at both the 5' and 3' site
ends of the viral DNA. The typical LTR (Figure 3)

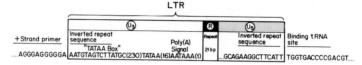

Structure RSV LTR

(H Varmus Science 216 812-820 1982)

FIGURE 3

contains a direct nucleotide sequence at the center which
is flanked on the 5' and 3' sites by U3 and U5 regions
containing inverted base sequences. The U3 component of
the LTR also contains the poly A signal for signaling the
viral RNA to be terminated with a long poly A repeat.
Further upstream in the 5' region is the TATAA box which
signals the initiation of transcription of the DNA to
hnRNA by the cellular polymerase. The structure of the
provirus in which terminal repeats enclose
protein-encoding genes shows a close similarity to the
general structure of genetic transport elements which have
been identified in bacteria and yeasts (Shimotohno et al.,
1980). This general structure has led Temin to propose
that retroviruses arose when a cellular gene coding for a
primitive reverse transcriptase became flanked on either
side by an LTR. The virus would then evolve by subsequent
capture of genes coding for gag and env regions of the
present retroviruses (Temin, 1980).

The analogy to genetic transport elements of bacteria
and yeasts suggests the use of retroviruses for the
deliberate construction of gene transporting vectors by
fusion of the LTR elements with DNA's coding for various
genes. Studies along these lines have already given
preliminary success (Shimotohno and Temin, 1981; Tabin
et al., 1982).

As shown in Figure 4, a composite plasmid vector in
which the Maloney leukemia virus has been integrated is
cleaved at bam sites and then ligated to a bam fragment
containing DNA coding for herpes simplex virus thymidine
kinase protein. The resulting plasmid can then be
infected into NIH3T3, thymidine kinase minus (TK$^-$) cells
and selected in HAT medium to give transformants that are
TK$^+$. In fact superinfection of these cells with Maloney
leukemia virus then leads to high titer virus stock in

which the thymidine kinase gene has been incorporated.
The Shimotohno-Temin studies have defined a number of
parameters that are necessary for construction of high
titers of these hybrid virions.

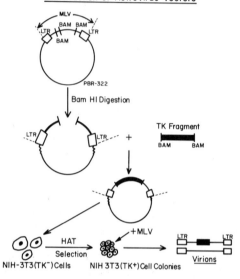

Construction of Retrovirus Vectors

[C J Tabin et al Mol.&Cell. Biol. 2, 426–436, 1982]

FIGURE 4

Production of mouse mammary tumor virus in infected
cells is stimulated by glucocorticoids (Ringold et al.,
1977). An important recent finding has been evidence that
the LTR region of mammary tumor virus is subject to
activation by complexes of steroids with hormone
receptors. The role of the LTR in this reaction has been
elucidated in the study of composite plasmids (Lee et al.,
1981). As shown in Figure 5 a composite plasmid of BR322

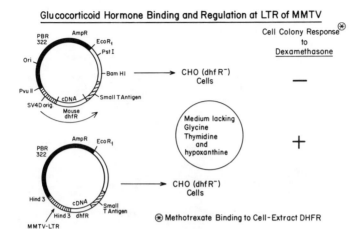

Glucocorticoid Hormone Binding and Regulation at LTR of MMTV

[F Lee et al Nature 294 228-232 1981]

FIGURE 5

and SV40 components (including SV40 origin) can be constructed, which can replicate in either bacterial or mammalian cells. Inserted into this PSV2 composite plasmid is the DNA coding for mouse dyhydrofolic acid reductase. This plasmid, on infection of Chinese hamster ovary cells which are deficient in hydrofolic acid reductase, transforms them into dyhydrofolic acid reductase positive cells. When these cells are, however, stimulated with dexamethasone there is not an increased yield of dyhydrofolic acid reductase. In contrast, a similar plasmid in which the promoter region of the SV40 has been removed and replaced with the LTR component of the mouse mammary tumor virus gives similar results on infection of Chinese hamster ovary cells, except that the cells are subject to dexamethasone stimulation of dyhydrofolic acid reductase.

It has recently been found that the SV40 DNA contains a region situated upstream from the origin which contains a tandem repeat of a 72 base pair DNA sequence and which appears vital for transcription of the early T antigens which are involved in transformation of cells by the SV40 virus. Recently Levinson and his associates have shown that the LTRs of retroviruses contain a functionally similar sequence (Levinson et al., 1982). This was done

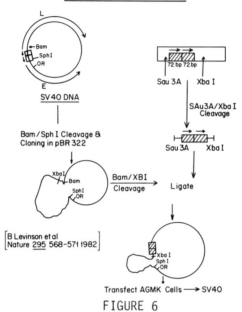

LTR Base Repeat Region as Replacement for
SV40 "Enhancing Elements"

FIGURE 6

(Fig. 6) by replacing the tandem 72 base pair repeat in
the SV40 DNA with a similar repeat unit excised from the
MSV-LTR and annealed into a composite plasmid. This
plasmid then, on infection of African green monkey cells,
produced infectious SV40 virus, whereas in the absence of
the 72 base pair repeat, the SV40 virus by itself was not
infectious.

It was earlier shown by the Varmus-Bishop group that
uninfected chicken cells typically produce only a few mRNA
copies of the cellular src onc. In contrast, cells
infected and transformed by the sarcoma viruses may
typically produce 100 or upwards mRNA copies of the
v-src. The role of the LTRs in activating either the
cellular or viral oncs has been demonstrated by the Vande
Woude group in studies in which they have examined intact
provirus and cellular or viral mos as existing alone or as
coupled to an LTR at the 5' or 3' positions (Oskarsson
et al., 1980). This they have done (Fig. 7) by
tranfecting 3T3 cells with the mos oncs, derived from the
virus or the cell, either alone or coupled to the

appropriate LTR. It will be noted that in this assay the
v–mos and c–mos or LTR elements are inactive in

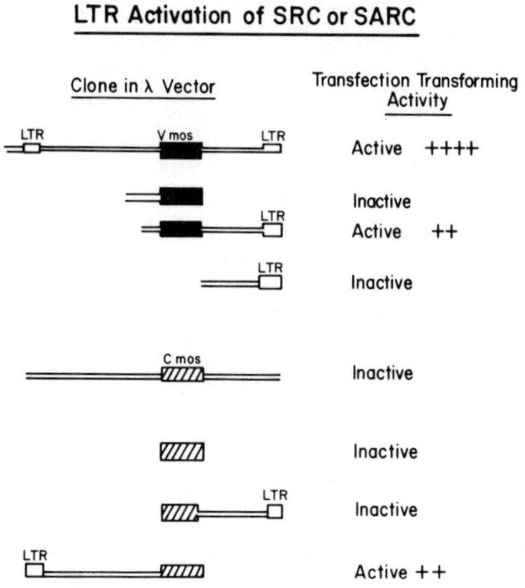

LTR Activation of SRC or SARC

Clone in λ Vector   Transfection Transforming
                                Activity

LTR   V mos   LTR   Active ++++

                              Inactive
                     LTR   Active   ++

                     LTR   Inactive

          C mos   Inactive

                               Inactive

                     LTR   Inactive

LTR   Active ++

[M. Oskarsson et al. Science 207 1222–1224 1980]

FIGURE 7

transfection of 3T3 cells. Likewise, the cellular mos
coupled with an LTR at the 3' end of the Moloney virus DNA
is also inactive, whereas the viral mos coupled at the 3'
end is moderately active. The c–mos DNA when ligated to
the bulk of the proviral DNA but minus the LTRs is also
inactive. On the other hand, the cellular mos coupled
with an LTR through the 5' end is active. These data
clearly show the role of the LTR, particularly in the 5'
position relative to the onc gene, in activating the onc
gene for transcription.

    Genes mediate their effects through protein products.
For a considerable period the protein products of onc
genes remained elusive. The following strategy was
finally utilized for the isolation of the src gene product
(Brugge and Erikson, 1977). The Schmidt–Ruppin strain of
Rous sarcoma virus containing the src gene was inoculated
into rabbits to produce tumors. Serum is then collected
from the xenogeneic hosts bearing thse tumors and used in
an immunoprecipitation reaction with extracts of
radioactively labelled cells infected with various strains

of the Schmidt-Ruppin virus. These virus strains include:
the Schmidt-Ruppin virus, temperature sensitive
Schmidt-Ruppin, a virus with a deletion mutant in the src
region, and an avian leukosis virus which does not contain
the src gene. Extracts of the cells were also exposed to
antisera against the various purified structural proteins
of the virus. The antisera then produced
immunoprecipitates which on treatment with sodium
dodecylsulfate and on electrophoretic separation on gels
permitted an identification of the unique protein
corresponding to the src gene. In more recent experiments
by Gilmer and Erickson the src gene has been incorporated
into a plasmid vector which has then been expressed in
E coli to produce the protein product (Gilmer and Erikson,
1981). The src gene and the viral onc genes of a number
of other viruses have been shown to yield phosphoproteins
that have kinase activity; that is the ability to transfer
phosphate groups. An intriguing feature of this kinase
activity is that the transfer is independent of cyclic AMP
and results in a transfer of the phosphate group from ATP
specifically to tyrosine on the recipient protein rather
than to serine as is usual in cyclic AMP-mediated
transfers (Hunter et al., 1980). Interestingly, when the
onc gene protein kinases are exposed to specific immune
sera the IgG in the immunoprecipitate is specifically
phosphorylated at the tyrosine residue. The
immunoprecipitates prepared by interaction of the
antiserum with extracts of transformed cells frequently
contain a cellular protein with a molecular weight of
53,000 (Brugge and Darrow, 1982). This same protein also
has been found in other transformed cell systems. Thus it
has been found bound to the middle T antigen of SV40
transformed cells (Linzer and Levine, 1979), in chemically
transformed cells (DeLeo et al., 1979), and bound to the
EBNA antigen produced on transformation of cells with the
Epstein-Barr virus (Luka et al., 1980). It should be
noted that Polyoma middle T antigen also possesses
tyrosine-specific kinase activity and is
membrane-associated (Turler, 1980). Examination of the
DNA base sequence of src gene (Czernilofsky et al., 1980)
has led to construction of amino acid sequence of the
60,000 molecular weight src protein product. This protein
has been shown to contain a hydrophobic region at the
amino terminus which is probably employed in anchorage to
the cell membrane and a more hydrophilic region containing
the kinase activity. This structure is in line with the

capacity of the pp60^{src} to bind to the cell membrane. This binding may be associated with physiological consequences, since it has been shown by Todaro and his associates that in cells transformed with the feline sarcoma virus epidermal growth factor (EGF) fails to bind to the EGF receptor (Todaro et al., 1976). This finding suggests that the presence of the src gene products in the cell membrane interferes with insulin-like activity. Cells transformed with acute transforming viruses in which the v-oncs contain phosphokinase activity also show elevated levels of phosphotyrosine (Hunter et al., 1980). The above findings indicate that a number of viral onc genes mediate their cell transformation effects through synthesis of specific proteins with tyrosine-specific and cyclic-AMP independent kinases, which then insert into the cell membrane and disrupt normal protein-hormonal control and skeletal protein phosphorylation. It should be noted that normal cells of several species express low levels of a protein homologous to pp60^{src} which is believed to be the product of the cellular c-onc (Opperman et al., 1979). The transformation event may therefore be one of dosage rather than the induction of a qualitatively unique protein. Of particular interest are the experiments of Scolnick and his group who have prepared monoclonal antibodies against onc gene product and have used these monoclonals to demonstrate heightened levels of the protein product in transformed cells. In contrast, cells transformed with a number of other acutely transforming viruses (e.g. the Maloney sarcoma virus containing v-mos or the Harvey sarcoma virus containing h-ras) do not show elevated phosphotyrosine levels. In this connection it is of interest that cells transformed by the Kirsten ras and also various human carcinoma cells express a protein with a lactic dehydrogenase activity (LDHk) which is inducible on oxygen deprivation (Anderson and Kovacik).

I have already briefly alluded to the transfection process in which 3T3 mouse cells can be infected with DNA from a variety of tumors of mouse or human origin and be morphologically transformed. Of great interest has been the finding that pathologically similar tumors derived from different individuals can yield DNA which transfects the 3T3 cells and that the DNA of these tumors shows a similar pattern of susceptibility to digestion with restriction enzymes. The experimental findings are that three different human bladder carcinomas show similar or

identical molecular lesions associated with their
neoplasias. Electrophoresis of these restriction
fragments and hybridization to the DNA of various oncs has
identified that the DNA rescued in this transfection
process corresponds to the Harvey ras (Parada et al.,
1982; Goldfarb et al., 1982). Thus in these experiments,
three different human neoplasias have been shown to be
associated with an identical onc gene. Similar
experiments on transfection of 3T3 cells with either
various mouse mammary carcinomas or human mammary
carcinomas indicate that the DNA employed in the
transfection shows a similar pattern of susceptibility to
restriction enzymes (Lane et al., 1981). Of great
interest has been the recent finding that either B-cell
leukemias or T-cell leukemias of the human can transfect
mouse 3T3 cells and that the pattern of susceptibility to
various restriction enzymes corresponds with the stage of
maturation of the cells along their respective lineages
(Lane et al., 1982). Taken as a whole, the above data
suggests that various neoplastic pathologies, of both man
and mouse, can be associated with transfection of specific
DNA sequences. Clearly, the further identification of
such sequences is of intense interest. These gratifying
results must however be viewed in the context of presently
existing difficulties. Transfection of approximately 50%
of human tumors fails to result in transformation of 3T3
cells. Furthermore, in some instances of 3T3 cell
transformation the active transfecting DNA is not
identifiable with the onc gene that appears to be
expressed actively in the tumor. Thus the myc gene is not
rescued from bursal lymphomas of fowl (Lane et al., 1982).

A number of mechanisms have already been elucidated by
which retroviruses produce pathology in the infected
host. Infection of an appropriate cell type with acute
transforming viruses (e.g. infection of fibroblast cells
with a virus containing a src gene or infection of
lymphoid precursor cells with a virus containing the abl
gene) can result in rapid cell transformations and the
expression of the specific malignant phenotypes. It must
be noted, however, that in studies to date the various onc
genes do not map contiguous to inserted proviruses, such
as EV-1 or EV-3 in the chicken. Furthermore, laboratory
studies have implied that the acutely infectious viruses
have arisen either through genetic recombination between
the retroviruses and an onc gene, either spontaneously or

in the laboratory (Hanafusa et al., 1977). Thus this mechanism may be relevant predominantly to laboratory infections with acutely transforming viruses. Perhaps of more importance to naturally occurring neoplasias is an understanding of the pathologies associated with the slow infectious retroviruses. Here two mechanisms of pathogenesis have already been defined. In one mechanism, that of the AKR mouse leukemia, a virus is inherited as a provirus but has intrinsically a very low capacity for production of disease. On activation in the host, however, and on spread through various tissues, it provides an opportunity for recombination with other proviruses which are defective either in the LTR or in the env gene regions. The result of this recombination is the internal production within the host of an acutely infectious transforming virus that has an altered tissue range as specified by the recombinant envelope (Hartley et al., 1977). This mechanism appears to be the predominant mechanism involved in the production of T-cell lymphomas of the mouse. In contrast, in the production of the B-cell leukemias of the chicken, it has been shown by appropriate restriction mapping that a common feature of pathogenesis is the deletion of the bulk of the viral elements and the insertion of a residual LTR in a 5' position relative to the c-myc of the fowl. This finding has been demonstrated by two different groups (Hayward et al., 1981; Payne et al., 1982). Of interest, however, is that a third group (Cooper and Neiman, 1981) finds a similar picture but also finds that on transfection of the DNA of these bursal lymphomas into 3T3 cells the myc gene is not transfected. Lastly, it should be noted that proviruses which are silent during the lifetime of the host (e.g. the ev locus of the chicken and MMTV provirus of the mouse) can be activated by events which result in demethylation of the LTR sequence of the virus.

Despite the great diligence of virologists the separate isolation by different groups of investigators of similar or identical retroviruses associated with adult T cell lymphomas (HTLV) provide the only widely accepted example of an infectious retrovirus implicated in a human neoplasia (Poiesz et al., 1981; Yoshido et al., 1982). The demonstration that HTLV is an exogenous infectious retrovirus (Robert-Guroff et al., 1982; Hinuma et al., 1981) clearly suggests careful evaluation of steps required to prevent its transmission in human populations. Success in isolation of HTLV will bring renewed zest to the search for other infectious retroviruses associated with other human cancers. Meanwhile the perspective of the virologist has enlarged to also include cognizance of proviruses; LTR's and moveable genetic elements; and onc genes and their potential capture by recombination with retroviruses and their activation by propinquity to LTR sequences. This new body of information is providing new insights into the molecular lesions associated with various neoplasias. We can reasonably expect that this new information should provide greater effectiveness to efforts for prevention, diagnosis and treatment of human cancer.

REFERENCES

Anderson GR, Kovacik WP (1981). LDH_k, an unusual oxygen-sensitive lactate dehydrogenase expressed in human cancer. Proc. Natl. Acad. Sci. 78:3209.

Breznik T, Cohen C (1982). Altered methylation of endo-genous viral promoter sequences during mammary carcino-genesis. Nature 295:255.

Brugge JS, Darrow D (1982). Rous sarcoma virus-induced phosphorylation of a 50,000-molecular weight cellular protein. Nature 295:250.

Brugge JS, Erikson RL (1977). Identification of a trans-formation specific antigen induced by an avian sarcoma virus. Nature 269:346.

Cooper GM, Neiman PE (1981). Two distinct candidate transforming genes of lymphoid leukosis virus-induced neoplasms. Nature 292:857.

Czernilofsky AP, Levinson AD, Varmus HE, Bishop JM, Tischer E, Goodman HM (1980). Nucleotide sequence of an avian sarcoma virus oncogene (SRC) and proposed amino acid sequence for gene product. Nature 287:198.

Davidson EH (1976). In "Gene Activity in Early Develop-ment", Second Edition, New York: Academic Press, p 2.

DeLeo AB, Jay G, Appella E, DuBois GC, Law LL, Old LL (1979). Detection of transformation related antigen in chemically induced sarcomas and other transformed cells of the mouse. Proc Natl Acad Sci USA 76:2420.

Gilmer TM, Erikson RL (1981). Rous sarcoma virus trans-forming protein p60SRC, expressed in E coli, functions as a protein kinase. Nature 294:771.

Goldfarb M, Shimizu K, Perucho M, Wigler M (1982). Isolation and preliminary characterization of a human transforming gene from T24 bladder carcinoma cells. Nature 296:404.

Groudine M, Eisenman R, Weintraub H (1981). Chromatin structure of endogenous retroviral genes and activation by an inhibitor of DNA methylation. Nature 292:311.

Hanafusa H, Halpern CC, Buchagen DL, Kawai S (1977). Recovery of avian sarcoma virus from tumors induced by transformation-defective mutants. J Exp Med 146:1735.

Hartley JW, Wolford NK, Old LJ, Rowe WP (1977). A new class of murine leukemia virus associated with the development of spontaneous lymphomas. Proc Natl Acad Sci USA 74:789.

Hayward WS, Neel BG, Astran SM (1981). Activation of a cellular onc gene by promoter insertion in an ALV-induced lymphoid leukosis. Nature 290:475.

Hinuma Y, Nagata K, Hanaoka M, Nakai M, Matsumoto T, Kimoshita KJ, Shirakawa S, Miyoshi I (1981). Adult T cell leukemia: Antigen in an ATL cell line and detection of antibodies to the antigen in human sera. Proc Natl Acad Sci USA 78:6476.

Hunter T, Sefton BM, Beemon K (1980). Phosphorylation of tyrosine: A mechanism of transformation shared by a number of otherwise unrelatred RNA tumor viruses. In "Animal Virus Genetics", Academic Press, p 499.

Jahner D, Stuhlmann H, Stewart CL, Harbers K, Lohler J, Simon I, Jaenisch R (1982). De Novo methylation and expression of retroviral genomes during mouse embryogenesis. Nature 298:623.

Lane MA, Sainten A, Cooper GM (1981). Activation of related transforming genes in mouse and human mammary carcinomas. Proc Natl Acad Sci USA 78:5185.

Lane MA, Sainten A, Cooper GM (1982). Stage-specific transforming genes of human and mouse B- and T-lymphocyte neoplasms. Cell 28:873.

Lee F, Mulligan R, Berg P, Ringold G (1981). Glucocorticoids regulate expression of dihydrofolate reductase cDNA in mouse mammary tumor virus chimaeric plasmids. Nature 294:228.

Levinson B, Khoury G, Vande Woude G, Gruss P (1982). Activation of the SV40 genome by 72 base pair tandem repeats of Molony sarcoma virus. Nature 295:568.

Linzer DJH, Levine AJ (1979). Characterization of a 54K Dalton cellular SV40 tumor antigen present in SV40 transferred cells and uninfected embryonal carcinoma cells. Cell 17:43.

Luka J, Jornvall H, Klein G (1980). Purification and biochemical characterization of the Epstein-Barr virus-determined nuclear antigen and an associated protein with a 53,000 Dalton subunit. J Virol 35:592.

Oppermann H, Levinson AD, Varmus HE, Levintow L, Bishop JM (1979). Uninfected vertebrate cells contain a protein that is closely related to the product of the avian sarcoma virus transforming gene (SRC). Proc Natl Acad Sci USA 76:1804.

Oskarsson M, McClements WL, Blair DG, Maizel JV, Vande Woude GF (1980). Properties of a normal mouse cell DNA sequence (sarc) homologous to the src sequence of Moloney Sarcoma Virus. Science 207:1222.

Parada LF, Tabin CJ, Shih C, Weinberg RA (1982). Human EV bladder carcinoma oncogene is homologue of Harvey sarcoma virus ras gene. Nature 297:474.

Payne GS, Bishop JM, Varmus HE (1982). Multiple arrangements of viral DNA and an activated host oncogene in bursal lymphomas. Nature 295:209.

Pierce GB (1972). Differentiation and cancer. In Harris R, Alin P, Viza D (eds): "Cell Differentiation", Munksgaard, Copenhagen, p 109.

Poiesz BJ, Ruscetti FW, Reitz MS, Kalyanaraman VS, Gallo RC (1981). Isolation of a new type C retrovirus (HTLV) in primary uncultured cells of a patient with Sezary T-cell leukemia. Nature 294:268.

Ringold GM,, Yamamoto KR, Bishop JM, Varmus HE (1977). Glucocorticoid-stimulated accumulation of mouse mammary tumor virus RNA: Increased rate of synthesis of viral RNA. Proc Natl Acad Sci USA 74:2879.

Robert-Guroff M, Nakao Y, Notake K, Ito Y, Sliski A, Gallo R (1982). Natural antibodies to human retrovirus HTLV in a cluster of Japanese patients with adult T cell leukemia. Science 215:975.

Shimotohno K, Temin HM (1981). Formation of infectious progeny virus after insertion of Herpes Simplex Thymidine Kinase Gene into DNA of an avian retrovirus. Cell 26:67.

Stehelin D, Varmus HE, Bishop JM, Vogt PK (1976). DNA related to the transforming gene(s) of avian sarcoma viruses is present in normal avian DNA. Nature 260:170.

Stockert E, Old LJ, Boyse EA (1971). The GIX System. A cell-surface alloantigen associated with murine leukemia virus; Implication regarding chromosomal integration of the viral genome. J Exp Med 133:1334.

Tabin CJ, Hoffmann JW, Goff SP, Weinberg RM (1982).
   Adaptation of a retrovirus as a eukaryotic vector
   transmitting the Herpes Simplex Virus Thymidine Kinase
   Gene. Mol Cell Biol 2:426.
Temin HM (1980). Origin of retroviruses from cellular
   moveable genetic elements. Cell 21:599.
Todaro GJ, DeLarco JE, Cohen S (1976). Transformation by
   murine and feline sarcoma viruses specifically blocks
   binding of epidermal growth factor to cells. Nature
   264:26.
Turler H (1980). The tumor antigens and the early functions of polyoma virus. Mol Cell Biochem 32:62.
Varmus HE (1982). Form and function of retroviral
   proviruses. Science 216:812.
Yoshida M, Miyoshi I, Hinuma Y (1982). Isolation and
   characterization of retrovirus from cell lines of human
   adult T-cell leukemia and its implication in the
   disease. Proc Natl Acad Sci USA 79:2031.

IDENTIFICATION AND CHARACTERIZATION OF ONCOGENES IN VARIOUS ANIMAL HOST SYSTEMS

Oncogenes and Retroviruses: Evaluation of Basic Findings and Clinical Potential, pages 23–35
© 1983 Alan R. Liss, Inc., 150 Fifth Avenue, New York, NY 10011

USING RETROVIRUSES AS INSERTIONAL MUTAGENS TO IDENTIFY CELLULAR ONCOGENES

Harold E. Varmus, M.D.

Department of Microbiology and Immunology

University of California, San Francisco 94143

SUMMARY

Three criteria have been used to identify cellular genes that might play a role in oncogenesis: (i) homology with known viral transforming genes (v-onc's); (ii) activated expression in tumor cells; and (iii) transforming activity in cultured mouse cells. We have been exploring the hypothesis that retroviruses lacking oncogenes activate cellular oncogenes by insertional mutagenesis. Our approach is to locate proviruses within the chromosomal DNA of clonal populations of tumor cells, and to identify activated transcriptional units in flanking cellular DNA. The central findings that have emerged from such studies in our laboratory and others indicate that: (i) insertion of avian leukosis virus (ALV) DNA can activate c-myc, a previously identified cellular homologue of a viral transforming gene, by various arrangements of proviral and c-myc DNA; (ii) most mammary carcinomas in C3H mice carry new mouse mammary tumor virus (MMTV) proviruses within an unidentified 20 kilobase region of the mouse genome that contains at least one activated transcriptional unit; (iii) proviruses of three viruses (ALV), chicken syncytial virus (CSV), and myeloblastosis-associated virus (MAV) are present in the c-myc locus in avian B cell lymphomas, suggesting that the same gene is activated during induction of a single type of tumor by different viruses; and (iv) MAV-induced nephroblastomas do not contain proviral insertions near c-myc, implying that the same virus may affect different genes in different types of tumor.

METHODS FOR IDENTIFYING PUTATIVE CELLULAR ONCOGENES

It has long been recognized that somatic and inherited
mutations are likely to be important in oncogenesis (Cairns
1980; Ponder 1980), but experimental access to the nature of
the affected genes has been gained only recently. There are
presently at least three different ways to identify cellular
genes that may be factors in oncogenic mechanisms and are
hence called "cellular oncogenes" (Fig 1).

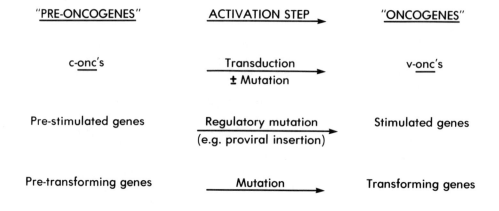

Figure 1. "Pre-oncogenes" are normal cellular genes of unknown function that can be activated in some of the indicated
ways to produce "oncogenes", as discussed in the text.

The first method depends upon the observation that the transforming genes of retroviruses are derived from cellular genes (Bishop 1981). Over 15 different viral oncogenes (v-onc's, in the nomenclature of Coffin et al 1981) have now been distinguished, and each is homologous to a cellular gene (c-onc) identified by molecular hybridization techniques (for review, see Bishop and Varmus 1982). All c-onc genes may be considered likely to have oncogenic potential, since they are closely related to viral transforming genes, but they are normally expressed at low levels, and only in a few instances has augmented expression been shown to render these genes competent to transform cultured cells (Blair et al 1981; De Feo et al 1981). Thus, during the transition of c-onc's to v-onc's, through a retroviral transduction process that is still poorly understood, the genes appear to be significantly mutated as well as placed under the control of a more potent transcriptional promoter. Similarly complex events might be necessary for c-onc's to play a role in oncogenesis, without retroviral transduction.

The second strategy for identification of putative cellular oncogenes depends upon the hypothesis that genes expressed at an abnormally high level in tumor cells might be involved in tumorigenesis. This is a particularly treacherous approach, since it is possible that cellular transformation provokes an extensive change in the cell's transcriptional program, particularly through epigenetic mechanisms; hence the enhanced expression of many genes may be the result, rather the cause, of the disordered behavior of the cell. However, when heightened expression is caused by mutations affecting the same locus in several tumors, it is probable that that locus is implicated in the oncogenic mechanism. Gene amplification, base substitutions within the transcriptional promoter, or gross rearrangements are among the kinds of mutation that could affect the level of expression. A particularly provocative approach, illustrated below in considerable detail, has been to seek genes whose activity is affected by insertional mutations involving retroviral proviruses. In these instances, the initiating event in tumorigenesis appears to be an insertion of proviral DNA, with its efficient regulatory apparatus, near a cellular oncogene. Since molecular probes for the mutagen (proviral DNA) are available, putative oncogenes can be identified and isolated by their linkage to the provirus.

The third means to identify putative cellular oncogenes

relies upon the use of DNA transformation procedures. Cultured mouse fibroblasts (NIH/3T3 cells) undergo morphological transformation when exposed to DNA from certain tumors
and tumor cell lines (Shih et al 1979; Cooper et al 1980).
Since DNA similarly prepared from normal cells is not
transforming in such assays, it is generally assumed that
the transforming activity reflects mutations that have altered either the expression or structural properties of a
cellular gene with oncogenic potential. It is uncertain
whether the mutated genes scored in this assay represent
primary or later events in the oncogenic process, particularly when the donor DNA is prepared from cultured tumor
cell lines rather than primary tumors. Furthermore, in many
cases, the assay succeeds despite profound differences of
species and tissue type between the donor and the indicator
cells. Nevertheless, the procedure represents a potent way
to identify cellular genes that have the documented capacity
to initiate oncogenic change in (at least) an established
cell line.

By identifying host-derived viral transforming genes
("v-onc's"), genes over-expressed in tumors ("stimulated
genes"), and genes in tumor DNA that transform NIH/3R3 cells
("transforming genes"), the scientific community has defined
three potentially overlapping sets of cellular genes (Figs 1
and 2). Under normal conditions, the members of each set
can be considered "pre-oncogenes", genes with the potential
to be converted to an oncogenic form by events that alter
the expression or substance of their products (Fig. 1). To
call such genes "pre-oncogenes" is not meant to imply that
their sole function is to await activation to oncogenic
status; on the contrary, the evolutionary conservation and
frequent low level expression of these genes bespeak important roles in cell growth or development.

ONCOGENES

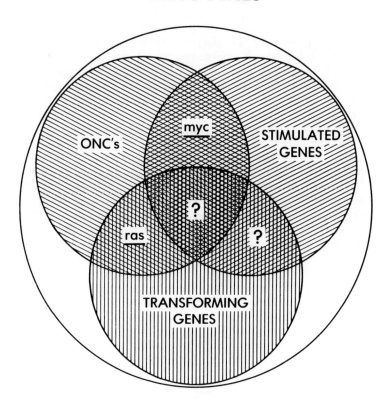

Figure 2. The figure illustrates overlaps among oncogenes detected by the three methods described in the text.

At the moment, it seems probable that the three experimental approaches can bring to our attention many, but not all, of the host genes involved in various forms of cancer. Other avenues---e.g., precise mapping of the affected loci in certain familial cancer syndromes (Ponder 1980)---may be necessary to allow identification of other members of the general class of cellular oncogenes (Fig 2). There is, on the other hand, the encouraging evidence that the three available strategies occasionaly detect the same genes; this suggests that the number of oncogenes is not unworkably large and that the three procedures---all unconventional from the viewpoint of a classical geneticist---may in some sense validate each other. To date, there are two genes--- c-myc and c-erb B---that have been encountered both as homologues of viral transforming genes and as cellular genes linked to tumor-inducing proviruses (Hayward et al 1981; T. Fung and H.J. Kung pers commun). Likewise, there are two genes (c-Ki-ras and c-Ha-ras), members of a complex gene family (Chang et al 1982), that have been isolated both as c-onc's and as transforming genes from murine and human tumors (Parada et al 1982; Der et al 1982; Santos et al 1982).

In this brief essay, I will review recent efforts in our laboratory and others to identify celllar oncogenes by their linkage to integrated viral DNA acting as a mutational agent to augment gene expression. Although DNA viruses, such as the human hepatitis B virus, can be envisioned to induce tumors by such mechanisms, positive findings have thus far been limited to retroviruses, and a few introductory comments about retroviral pathogenesis will facilitate subsequent discussion.

V-ONC VIRUSES AND INSERTIONAL MUTAGENESIS

The pathological spectrum of retroviruses is vast (see Teich et al 1982), but tumorigenic viruses can be conveniently placed in two categories: those viruses that carry onc genes transduced from normal cells, and those that contain only sequences implicated in viral replication. Two general hypotheses have received the most attention as explanations for the oncogenic activity of v-onc viruses: that some component of the viral genome may serve as an oncogene, although it is not derived from cellular genes, as are conventional onc sequences, and that proviruses may act as mutational agents, thereby affecting the behavior of host genes.

Retroviruses could instigate mutations in infected cells in several ways. As agents that introduce their genomes more or less randomly into host chromosomes, they are capable of inactivating host genes by interrupting them. This capacity is exemplified by the insertional mutations produced by murine leukemia virus (MLV) proviruses that have been integrated within a Rous sarcoma virus (RSV) provirus responsible for the transformed phenotype of the host (Varmus et al 1981). An insertional mutation is also apparently responsible for the dilute coat-color allele in certain inbred mouse strains (Jenkins et al 1981). However, mutations that inactivate genes are likely to be recessive lesions, and the target gene for an oncogenic mutation of this type would have to be sex-linked or inactivated on both autosomal chromosomes to produce the tumor phenotype. A more promising possibility is that a provirus would activate the expression of host genes, particularly genes adjacent to the integration site through the agency of viral regulatory signals encoded in long terminal repeats (LTRs; see Varmus, 1982, for review). Such lesions would be dominant in most cases, permitting a single insertion to induce a tumor. Lastly, retroviruses might stimulate the host's own mutational mechanisms to yield any of the various genetic changes that have been implicated in neoplasia (see, for example, Cairns 1980).

LYMPHOMAGENESIS BY AVIAN LEUKOSIS VIRUS

Of the tumors induced by v-onc viruses, avian B cell lymphomas have probably been the most informative mechanistically and serve as the paradigm for insertional mechanisms in neoplasia. These tumors arise in certain susceptible lines of chickens 6-12 months after newborn animals have been inoculated with various strains of avian leukosis virus (ALV). During the preneoplastic stage, large numbers of cells in the target organ, the bursa of Fabricius, become infected, as evidenced by the introduction of ALV DNA into different sites in the genomes of many cells. Analysis of virus-specific DNA from tumors reveals a pattern consistent with the clonal origin of the tumor cells: Proviral DNA appears to be in the same site in most or all of the cells (Neiman et al 1980; Payne et al 1981; Neel et al 1981; Fung et al 1981). All tumors that have been examined in this

fashion retain at least a part of one provirus, suggesting
that proviral DNA is important for maintenance of the tumor
phenotype; however, several tumors contain only proviral DNA
afflicted by deletions and not expressed at detectable levels (Payne et al 1981; Neel et al 1981), implying that products of viral genes are not necessary to maintain tumorous
growth. The experiments of Neel et al (1981) and Payne et
al (1981) further demonstrated that the ALV proviruses, even
the defective ones, were able to stimulate transcription of
flanking host DNA; mapping experiments suggested that the
flanking sequences might be the same in several tumors. Using annealing reagents available for several onc sequences,
Hayward et al (1981) then showed that the insertion site in
most tumors was within or adjacent to the c-myc locus and
that cells with interrupted loci contained elevated levels
of c-myc RNA. Meanwhile, Cooper and Neiman (1980) had
found that DNA from similar tumors was able to transform
NIH/3T3 cells; however, the transforming component appeared
to be separate from either ALV DNA or from the interrupted
c-myc domains (Cooper and Neiman 1981).

The following sequence of events could produce the
phenomena described in the preceding paragraph: (i) The oncogenic process is initiated in one of the rare ALV-infected
B cells that acquires a provirus near a c-myc locus, provided that the inserted DNA is suitably placed to enhance expression of c-myc and that the host cell is at a stage susceptible to the oncogenic consequences of heightened expression; (ii) development of the tumor phenotype requires additional genetic events, one of which is reflected in the
transforming activity of tumor DNA; and (iii) outgrowth of
tumorigenic clones is favored by mutations (e.g., deletions)
that affect the ability of proviral DNA to enhance c-myc expression or to direct synthesis of viral antigens to which
the host immune system is responsive. These conjectures
raise an additional series of questions: What is responsible
for the enhanced expression of c-myc? Are similar oncogenic
mechanisms operative in other tumors induced by v-onc
viruses? If so, what are the determinants of the oncogenic
spectra of various viruses? Can this approach be used to
identify new cellular oncogenes, including genes important
in human tumors and in tumors arising in the absence of
viruses?

HOW DO PROVIRUSES ENHANCE EXPRESSION OF ONCOGENES?

Most of the B-cell lymphomas examined to date exhibit
an arrangement of ALV DNA and c-myc conducive to the use of
a viral promoter for efficient transcription of the c-myc
gene (Hayward et al 1981). In these tumors, proviral DNA is
positioned on the 5' side of the two well-defined exons of
c-myc, in the same transcriptional orientation; because the
long terminal repeat (LTR) at the 5' end of proviral DNA is
often deleted or inactivated, the 3' LTR is presumed to provide the initiation site for transcription, producing abundant species with viral sequences linked to c-myc sequences
(Hayward et al 1981; Payne et al 1982). In several of the
tumors in our collection, however, proviral DNA is found on
the 5' side of c-myc, but in the opposite transcriptional
orientation (Payne et al 1982). We have also examined one
tumor in which part of an ALV provirus is present on the 3'
side of c-myc in the same transcriptional orientation (Payne
et al 1982). The residual LTR appears to provide the polyadenylation site for the abundant c-myc RNA; however,
again, the mechanism for enhanced expression is unknown,
although a similar situation has been generated by in vitro
ligation of an LTR to the 3' side of a cloned v-onc gene
(Blair et al 1980). It seems likely, based upon these unexpected arrangements of viral DNA and c-myc, that LTRs confer
upon adjacent regions of the chromosome the property of being transcribed efficiently from normally used or novel promoters. This property could depend upon the topology of the
local domain of DNA, upon the arrangement of chromatin proteins, or upon concentrations of RNA polymerase along the
chromosome.

EVIDENCE FOR INSERTIONAL MUTATION DURING ONCOGENESIS
BY MOUSE MAMMARY TUMOR VIRUS (MMTV)

MMTV lacks onc sequences and induces mammary adenocarcinomas derived from only one or a few of the many infected
cells in the preneoplastic gland (Cohen et al 1979). Furthermore, the tumors arise after considerable latency (the animals are usually infected shortly after birth by virus in
milk), and the DNA from tumors has been reported to
transform NIH/3T3 cells (Lane et al 1981). To determine the
role of the viral genome in mammary tumorigenesis, we identified a tumor in C3H mice that contained only one MMTV provirus, in addition to the proviruses endogenous to the germ

line. We cloned the 3' third of this provirus with about 15 kilobases (kb) of flanking cellular DNA, prepared probes for unique-sequence DNA from over 30 kb of the flanking region retrieved from a library of normal mouse DNA, and examined DNA from additional tumors (most bearing multiple new proviruses) for evidence of insertions in the same chromosomal domain (Nusse and Varmus, submitted for publication). In this survey, 18 of 26 tumors in C3H mice were found to contain MMTV proviruses within a region of 20 kb, a frequency much too high to be explained by chance.

These results encourage the view that the site of proviral integration is an important determinant in neoplasia by MMTV, since there is apparently a strong selection for the rare cell with an insertion in the chromosomal site we have isolated. Moreover, we have found that a polyadenylated species of RNA is present in the few tumors tested to date, but not in normal mammary glands. However, the identity of this transcriptional unit and chromosomal domain is not known. We have tested a large portion of the cloned chromosomal DNA for homology with about a dozen onc sequences thus far without positive results. Interestingly, DNA from MMTV-induced tumors, like most from ALV-induced bursal lymphomas, transforms 3T3 cells, and again the transforming activity does not appear to be closely linked to proviral DNA (Lane et al 1981).

WHAT IS THE RELATIONSHIP OF VIRUSES, INSERTION SITES, AND TUMOR TYPE?

Many retroviruses can induce multiple varieties of tumors, closely related retroviruses often cause tumors in different organs, and unrelated viruses appear responsible for the same type of tumor (Gross 1970; Teich et al 1982). Although such phenomena are not yet understood, it is now possible to ask whether different v-onc⁻ viruses cause a single type of tumor by a single mechanism, and whether the same virus uses a single mechanism to produce tumors in different organs. For example, two v-onc⁻ viruses other than ALV have been found to produce insertional mutations in c-myc during the induction of B-cell lymphomas. Several tumors induced in chickens by the chicken syncytial virus (CSV), a reticuloendotheliosis virus unrelated to ALV, show evidence of proviral insertions near c-myc, deletions affecting cellular and perhaps proviral DNA, and sometimes am-

plification of the interrupted c-myc locus (Noori-Daloii et
al 1982). Lymphomas produced in quail by myeloblastosis-
associated virus-1 (MAV-1), a virus differing from ALV principally in the LTR domain, also contain insertions of MAV-
specific DNA adjacent to c-myc (D. Westaway and C. Moscovici, unpublished results). Although c-myc RNA was not measured in these two instances, it seems likely that three different viruses - ALV, CSV, and MAV - initiate B-cell lymphomagenesis by an insertional activation of c-myc.

On the other hand, we have examined DNA from over a
dozen renal tumors, mainly nephroblastomas, induced by MAV
strains, and have failed to observe any disruptions of the
c-myc locus (D. Westaway and C. Moscovici, unpublished
results). Thus, very similar or identical viruses appear to
employ different mechanisms to cause tumors in different organs. The integration site (or sites) occupied by MAV DNA
in the renal tumors has yet to be identified.

ACKNOWLEDGMENTS

Work in this laboratory is supported by grants Nos. CA
19287, CA 12705 and CA 09043 from the National Institutes of
Health and MV 481 from the American Cancer Society. This
manuscript is a revised version of a paper to appear in the
1982 M.D. Anderson Symposium.

REFERENCES

Bishop JM, Varmus HE (1982). Functions and origins of retro-
viral transforming genes. In Weiss R, Teich N, Varmus HE,
Coffin J (eds.): "Molecular Biology of Tumor Viruses
Part III RNA Tumor Viruses," New York: Cold Spring Harbor
Press, p 999.
Blair DG, McClements WL, Oskarsson MK, Fischinger PJ, Vande
Woude GF (1980). Biological activity of cloned Moloney
sarcoma virus DNA: Terminally redundant sequences may
enhance transformation efficiency. Proc Nat Acad Sci USA.
777:3504.
Cairns J (1980). The origins of human cancers. Nature
289:353.
Chang EH, Gonda MA, Ellis RW, Scolnick EM, Lowy DR (1982).
Human genome contains four genes homologous to transforming
genes of Harvey and Kirsten murine sarcoma viruses. Proc

Nat Acad Sci USA 79:4848.

Coffin JM, Varmus HE, Bishop JM, Essex M, Hardy WD, Martin GS, Rosenberg NE, Scolnick EM, Weinberg R, Vogt PK (1981). A proposal for naming host cell-derived inserts in retrovirus genomes. J Virol 40:953.

Cohen JC, Shank P, Morris VL, Cardiff R, Varmus HE (1979). Integration of the DNA of mouse mammary tumor virus in virus-infected normal and neoplastic tissues of the mouse. Cell 16:333.

Cooper GM, Neiman PE (1980). Transforming genes of neoplasms induced by avian lymphoid leukosis viruses. Nature 287:659.

Cooper GM, Neiman PE (1981). Two distinct candidate transforming genes of lymphoid leukosis virus-induced neoplasms. Nature 292:857.

Cooper GM, Okenquist S, Silverman L (1980). Transforming activity of DNA of chemically transformed and normal cells. Nature 284:418.

Der CJ, Krontiris TG, Cooper GM (1982). Transforming genes of human bladder and lung carcinoma cell lines are homologous to the ras genes of Harvey and Kirsten sarcoma viruses. Proc Nat Acad Sci USA 79:3637.

Fung YKT, Fadly AM, Crittenden LB, Kung HJ (1981). On the mechanism of retrovirus-induced avian lymphoid leukosis: Deletion and interpretation of the proviruses. Proc Nat Acad Sci USA 78:3418.

Gross L (1970). "Oncogenic Viruses." New York: Pergamon Press.

Hayward WS, Neel BG, Astrin SM (1981). Activation of a cellular onc gene by promoter insertion in ALV-induced lymphoid leukosis. Nature 290:475.

Jenkins NA, Copeland NG, Taylor BA, Lee BK (1981). Dilute (d) coat colour mutation of DBA/2J mice is associated with the site of integration of an ecotropic MuLV genome. Nature 293:370.

Lane MA, Sainten A, Cooper GM (1981). Activation of related transforming genes in mouse and human mammary carcinomas. Proc Nat Acad Sci USA 78:5185.

Neel BG, Hayward WS, Robinson HL, Fang J, Astrin SM (1981). Avian leukosis virus-induced tumors have common proviral integration sites and synthesize discrete viral RNAs: Oncogenesis by promoter insertion. Cell 23:323.

Neiman P, Payne LN, Weiss RA (1980). Viral DNA in bursal lymphomas induced by avian leukosis viruses. J Virol 34:178.

Noori-Daloii MR, Swift RA, Kung HI, Crittenden LB, Witter RL (1981). Sporatic integration of REV proviruses in avian bursal lymphomas. Nature 294:574.

Parada LF, Tabin CJ, Shih C, Weinberg RA (1982). Human EJ
bladder carcinoma oncogene is homologue of Harvey sarcoma
virus ras gene. Nature 297:474.
Payne GS, Bishop JM, Varmus HE (1982). Multiple arrangements
of viral DNA and an activated host oncogene in bursal lymphomas. Nature 295:209.
Payne GS, Courtneidge SA, Crittenden LB, Fadly AM, Bishop JM,
Varmus HE (1981). Analysis of avian leukosis virus DNA and
RNA in bursal tumors: Viral gene expression is not required
for maintenance of the tumor state. Cell 23:311.
Ponder B-J (1980). Genetics and cancer. Biochim Biophys Act
Revs on Cancer 605:369.
Santos E, Tronick SR, Aaronson SA, Pulciani S, Barbacid M
(1982). T24 human bladder carcinoma oncogene is an
activated form of the normal human homologue of BALB- and
Harvey-MSV transforming genes. Nature 298:343.
Shih C, Shilo B-Z, Goldfarb MP, Dannenberg A, Weinberg RA
(1979). Passage of phenotypes of chemically transformed
cells via transfection of DNA and chromatin. Proc Nat
Acad Sci USA 76:5714.
Teich N, Bernstein A, Mak T, Wyke J, Hardy W (1982). Retro-
viral diseases. In Weiss R, Teich N, Varmus HE, Coffin J
(eds.): "Molecular Biology of Tumor Viruses Part III RNA
Tumor Viruses," New York: Cold Spring Harbor Press, p 785.
Varmus HE, Quintrell N, Ortiz S (1981). Retroviruses as
mutagens: Insertion and excision of a nontransforming pro-
virus alter expression of a resident transforming provirus.
Cell 25:23.
Varmus HE (1982). Form and function of retroviral proviruses.
Science 216:812.

Oncogenes and Retroviruses: Evaluation of Basic Findings
and Clinical Potential, pages 37–42
© 1983 Alan R. Liss, Inc., 150 Fifth Avenue, New York, NY 10011

CANCER INDUCTION BY INSERTIONAL MUTAGENESIS: THE ROLE OF
VIRAL GENES IN AVIAN LEUKOSIS VIRUS INDUCED CANCERS.

H. L. Robinson[1], J. M. Coffin[2], P. N. Tsichlis[3],

P. R. Shank[4], P. Schatz[5], and L. Jensen[1]

[1]Worcester Foundation for Experimental Biology
Shrewsbury, MA 20420

[2]Dept. of Molecular Biology and Microbiology
Tufts University School of Medicine
Boston, MA 02111

[3]National Cancer Institute
Bethesda, MD 20205

[4]Brown University
Providence, RI 02912

[5]Massachusetts Institute of Technology
Cambridge, MA 02139

We have been using recombinants of avian leukosis
viruses to study the genetic basis of non-acute avian leukosis virus induced cancers (Robinson et al., 1980; 1982).
Avian leukosis viruses that induce non-acute disease are
replication competent viruses that have the genetic composition 5' U5, gag, pol, env, U3-3'. Gag, pol and env encode
the core antigens, RNA-directed DNA polymerase, and envelope glycoproteins, of the mature virion. U5 and U3 are
non-protein coding sequences that form the long terminal
repeat sequences (LTRs) of integrated proviral DNA. U3
encodes sequences implicated in transcriptional control of
eukaryotic genes. Actual transcription of retroviral mRNAs
is initiated at the left-hand boundary of U5.

In a typical oncogenicity test 10^6 infectious units of a relevant virus or recombinant virus are inoculated intravenously into day-old K28 chickens. At one month, a time by which chickens appear to be maximally viremic, spread of virus in the chickens is monitored by testing the sera of infected birds for particulate reverse transcriptase. Birds are then maintained in separate isolation and observed for tumor development out to one year of age. Birds that display signs of cancers are sacrificed. Tumors are harvested for histological analyses, biochemical analyses, and for recovery of virus.

Although our oncogenicity tests are remarkably simple in design, the chickens that we have bred for these tests and the viruses we have selected for these tests have resulted in experiments that have provided unique insights into the genetics of non-acute disease. K28 chickens have been bred for susceptibility to subgroup E avian leukosis viruses (Robinson and Lamoreux, 1976). Subgroup E avian leukosis viruses are carried in the germ line of chickens as proviral DNA. These viruses do not appear to be oncogenic (Motta et al., 1975). Our oncogenicity tests have then been carried out using viruses with subgroup E envelope antigens. Since our infecting viruses have the same envelope antigens as the endogenous viruses of chickens, our test system minimizes formation and spread of recombinants between the infecting virus and endogenous viruses. Any recombinant that is formed has the same host range as the infecting virus. The spread of such a recombinant is interfered with by the already established infection of the test virus. Routine oligonucleotide mapping of viruses recovered from tumors (two to four tumors per oncogenicity test) have displayed only the oligonucleotide markers of the virus that was used in the infection. Ours is the only system for the oncogenicity testing of retroviruses in their natural host that essentially eliminates obfuscation of the results by the formation and spread of viruses that are recombinants of the test virus and endogenous viruses.

The oncogenic parents of our first series of recombinants were helper viruses isolated from stocks of Bryan Rous sarcoma viruses. These viruses designated Rous associated viruses (RAVs) cause a high incidence of lymphoma and a low incidence of diseases such as adenocarcinomas, chondrosarcomas, osteopetrosis and nephroblastomas. The oncogenic parent of our second series of experiments was

Prague Rous sarcoma virus-B (PrRSV-B). Src deletion mutants of PrRSV-B cause a high incidence of osteopetrosis between two and five months after infection and a low incidence of lymphomas, chondrosarcomas, fibrosarcomas and adenocarcinomas. Thus the parents of our recombinant viruses exhibited three distinct phenotypes: (1) the ability to induce a relatively high incidence of lymphoma between three and ten months after infection, (2) the ability to induce a relatively high incidence of osteopetrosis between two and five months after infection and (3) the ability to induce a low incidence of a variety of cancers.

The first oncogenicity test we performed was designed to test whether or not the lymphomogenic potential of RAV-1 and RAV-2 were encoded in env. The recombinants we used to test the role of env in lymphomogenesis were a kind gift of Drs. T. and H. Hanafusa. These viruses, designated RAV-60s, were subgroup E recombinants of RAV-1 (subgroup A) or RAV-2 (subgroup B) with the endogenous viruses (subgroup E) that reside at the chromosomal loci ev 3 or ev 9. K28 chickens inoculated with RAV-60s developed the same incidence of lymphoma as chickens inoculated with RAV-1 (Robinson et al., 1980). This experiment was the first clear cut demonstration that envelope antigens do not determine the lymphomogenic potential of avian leukosis viruses. Until this time it had been hypothesized that viruses with subgroup E envelope antigens did not cause disease because of their envelope antigens.

The second series of oncogenicity tests was undertaken to dtermine the role of non env viral sequences in oncogenesis. In these experiments we used non-transforming subgroup E (NTRE) viruses that were recombinants of RAV-0 (a non-oncogenic virus encoded by the endogenous provirus that resides at ev 2), and PrRSV-B. RAV-0 and PrRSV-B were chosen as parents for this series of experiments because of their highly distinctive oligonucleotide markers (Coffin et al., 1978). The oligonucleotides that were unique to each of these viruses could be used to identify regions of the recombinant viral genomes that were of PrRSV-B or RAV-0 origin (Tsichlis and Coffin, 1980). Of the many NTRE recombinants isolated by Dr. Tsichlis, NTRE-2 and NTRE-7 were chosen for oncogenicity testing. NTRE-7 contained oligonucleotide markers of its oncogenic parent only in U3. By contrast, NTRE-2 contained two blocks of oligonucleotide markers of PrRSV-B, one in gp37, U3 and a second in gag, pol. RAV-0,

tdPr-B (the non-transforming src deletion of PrRSV-B),
NTRE-2,and NTRE-7 were inoculated into day-old K28 chickens.
The tdPr-B infected chickens developed a high incidence of
osteopetrosis between two and five months of infection and a
low incidence of other disease. RAV-0 did not cause disease.
Quite interestingly, NTRE-7 caused only a low incidence of a
variety of cancers late in infection: lymphomas, chondrosarcomas, osteopetrosis, nephroblastomas, and fibrosarcomas
(Robinson et al., 1982). In contrast NTRE-2 caused a relatively high incidence of early osteopetrosis as well as a
low incidence of a variety of cancers (Robinson et al., in
preparation). On the basis of this experiment, we suggest
that viral U3 sequences determine the potential of a virus
to induce a low incidence of a variety of cancers and that
sequences in gag, pol or in gp37, U3 determine the ability
of a virus to induce a high incidence of osteopetrosis.

We are currently examining the oncogenic potential of
viruses recovered from molecularly cloned DNAs and recombinants of these molecularly cloned DNAs. For this series of
experiments NY203 was cloned into the sac 1 site of lambda
Charon 16A and NTRE-2 was cloned into the sal 1 site of
lambda Charon 27. The two lambda clones were isolated by
Peter Schatz in Dr. Peter Shank's laboratory. Viruses recovered from the molecularly cloned DNAs appear to have the
same oncogenic potential as their biological parents. In
order to examine the role of gag-pol and gp37 LTR regions in
oncogenesis; sac-sal (gag-pol gp85) and sal-sac (gp37 LTR)
recombinants of NY203 and NTRE-2 have been constructed by
Peter Schatz, Lauren Jensen, and Dr. Shank in Dr. Shank's
laboratory. Duplicates of these recombinants are currently
being tested for their oncogenic potential in K28 chickens.
The chickens infected with two viruses containing the
gag-pol gp85 fragment of NTRE-2 and the gp37 LTR fragment of
NY203 but not chickens infected with the reciprocal recombinant are developing a high incidence of osteopetrosis. We
are still too early in the tests to see lymphomas. The
results to date, however, indicate that gag-pol sequences
determine whether or not a virus induces a high incidence of
osteopetrosis.

In summary our oncogenicity tests have indicated that
envelope genes do not encode the oncogenic potential of
avian leukosis viruses. Rather, of the three phenotypes we
are studying: potential to produce a low incidence of a
variety of diseases, potential to induce a high incidence of

lymphoma, and potential to induce a high incidence of osteopetrosis; our tests indicate that 1) the induction of a low
incidence of a variety of diseases is encoded by viral U3
sequences and that, 2) the induction of a high incidence of
osteopetrosis is encoded by viral gag-pol sequences.

Avian leukosis virus induced lymphomas result from insertional mutagenesis of the cellular gene c-myc (Hayward
et al., 1981; Payne et al., 1981) and avian leukosis virus
induced erythroblastosis results from insertional mutagenesis of the cellular gene c-erb (H. J. Kung and T. Fung,
personal communication, unpublished observations). Cancer
induction following insertional mutation of both myc and erb
selects for proviruses that cause overexpression of c-myc
or c-erb. The U3 sequences of the non-oncogenic virus RAV-0
contain transcriptional control elements that appear to be
about 10-fold less active than those present in the U3
sequences of oncogenic avian leukosis viruses (Hayward, 1977;
Wang et al., 1977). RAV-0 undergoes efficient integration
into chromosomal DNA of chicken cells. Thus the lack of
disease in RAV-0 infected chickens cannot be attributed to
the inability of RAV-0 to insert itself into chicken chromosomal DNA. Rather, cancer induction by non-acute avian leukosis viruses may require not only insertion of a provirus
adjacent to a potentially oncogenic cellular gene but the
ability of the inserted provirus to encode "overexpression"
of the adjacent oncogene.

The mapping of the osteopetrotic potential of viruses
to the gag-pol region of the genome is an interesting
result. The molecular basis of osteopetrosis is not defined
and osteopetrosis, in contrast to lymphoma, may in fact be
a non-malignant disease. Needless to say, it will be
extremely interesting to determine if avian leukosis virus
induced osteopetrosis, as lymphomas, results from insertional mutation of a host gene and if the lymphomogenic potential of avian leukosis virus, as the osteopetrogenic potential, maps to gag-pol.

Coffin JM, Champion M, Chabot F (1978). Nucleotide sequence
   relationships between the genomes of an endogenous and an
   exogenous avian tumor virus. J Virol 28:972.
Hayward WS (1977). Size and genetic content of viral RNAs
   in avian oncovirus infected cells. J Virol 24:47.
Hayward WS, Neel BG, Astrin SM (1981). ALV-induced lymphoid leukosis: activation of a ce-lular onc gene by

promoter insertion. Nature 290:475.

Motta JV, Crittenden LB, Purchase HG, Stone HA, Okazaki W, Witter RL (1975). Low oncogenic potential of avian endogenous RNA tumor virus infection or expression. J Nat Can Inst 55:685.

Payne GS, Bishop JM, Varmus HE (1981). Multiple arrangements of viral DNA and an activated host oncogene (c-myc) in bursal lymphomas. Nature 295:209.

Robinson HL, Lamoreux WF (1976). Expression of endogenous ALV antigens and susceptibility to subgroup E ALV in three stains of chickens. Virol 69:50.

Robinson HL, Pearson MN, DeSimone DW, Tsichlis PN, Coffin JM (1979). Subgroup E avian leukosis virus associated disease in chickens. Cold Spring Harbor Symp Quant Biol XLIV:1133.

Robinson HL, Blais BM, Tsichlis PN, Coffin JM (1982). At least two regions of the viral genome determine the oncogenic potential of avian leukosis viruses. PNAS 79:1225.

Tsichlis PN, Coffin JM (1980). Recombinants between endogenous and exogenous avian tumor viruses: role of the c region and other portions of the genome in the control of replication and transformation. J Virol 33:238.

Wang SV, Hayward WS, Hanafusa H (1977). Genetic variation in the RNA transcripts of endogenous virus genes in uninfected chicken cells. J Virol 24:64.

Oncogenes and Retroviruses: Evaluation of Basic Findings
and Clinical Potential, pages 43–56
© 1983 Alan R. Liss, Inc., 150 Fifth Avenue, New York, NY 10011

THE ORGANIZATION OF c-rel IN CHICKEN AND TURKEY DNAS

K.C. Wilhelmsen, I.S.Y. Chen[*] and H.M. Temin

McArdle Laboratory for Cancer Research
University of Wisconsin
Madison, WI 53706

[*]Present address
Division Hematology/Oncology
UCLA School of Medicine
Los Angeles, CA 90024

Weakly oncogenic retroviruses are competent for replication and produce tumors in infected animals only after long latency periods and with low efficiency. Highly oncogenic retroviruses are derived from weakly transforming retroviruses and contain additional sequences, called oncogenes, which enable them to cause tumors after a short latency period with high efficiency. Oncogenes have been transduced by weakly oncogenic retroviruses from cells which they have infected. The cellular sequences which have been transduced from the genomes of cells are called proto-oncogenes (Bishop and Varmus 1982).

Proto-oncogenes, c-oncs, are involved in two different evolutionary processes. The first process is evolutionary change of a proto-oncogene in a population and between two species. The second process is transduction of proto-oncogene sequences by a weakly oncogenic retrovirus. The consequence of this transduction is a dramatic alteration of phenotype caused by the transduced sequences from non-oncogenic to oncogenic. In this study we have examined the effect of these two processes on the structure of the proto-oncogene, c-rel.

REV-T

In our laboratory we have been studying reticulo-endotheliosis virus strain T (Rev-T). Rev-A is the helper virus associated with Rev-T and supplies helper functions in trans for those functions which have been deleted from Rev-T (Breitman et al. 1980; Gonda et al. 1980; Chen et al. 1981; Hu et al. 1981). Rev-A is probably a reasonable approximation of the weakly oncogenic parental virus that gave rise to Rev-T. Rev-T is an avian reticuloendotheliosis virus and contains the oncogene v-rel. v-rel is in Rev-T substituting for sequences which encode env in REV-A. In addition, Rev-T has a deletion relative to REV-A of nucleotide sequences which in the parental virus code for much of gag and pol (Rice et al. 1982; Chen et al. 1981). This deletion of sequences found in the parental virus is necessary for the expression of the full transforming potential of Rev-T (Chen and Temin 1982).

Rev-T was isolated from a tumor-bearing turkey in 1958 (Theilen et al. 1966). It is assumed that Rev-T arose when a weakly oncogenic reticuloendotheliosis virus infected a turkey cell and transduced a proto-oncogene homologous to v-rel. The cellular sequences which were transduced by Rev-T are called c-rel.

To study the organization of Rev-T, we first obtained a molecular clone of a Rev-T provirus. A recombinant DNA phage library was constructed with DNA from a turkey embryo acutely infected with Rev-T after partial digestion with EcoRI and size selection. One molecular clone of a transforming Rev-T provirus (Ch4A Rev-T 52B) was obtained. We previously obtained a molecular clone of a provirus of a weakly oncogenic reticuloendotheliosis virus strain A (Rev-A) in a similar manner (Chen et al. 1981). Fig. 1 shows restriction enzyme cleavage maps of Rev-A and Rev-T DNAs.

c-rel (turkey)

To clone the c-rel proto-oncogene sequences, we constructed recombinant DNA bacteriophage libraries from DNA prepared from fibroblasts of a turkey embryo (turkey 7) (Blattner et al. 1977; Karn et al. 1980). Recombinant phage were screened for clones that contain c-rel

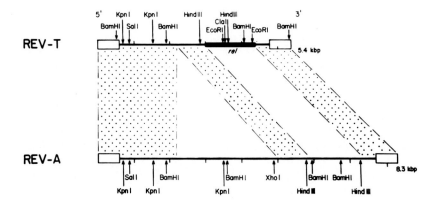

Fig. 1. DNA of Rev-T and Rev-A
     The restriction enzyme cleavage site maps of the
Rev-T and Rev-A portion of inserts of λCh4A Rev-T 52B and
2-20-6 (Rev-A) (Chen <u>et al</u>. 1981) are diagrammed above.
The LTR sequences are drawn as boxes, and the <u>rel</u> region
is drawn as a thick line.   The regions of homology
between Rev-A and Rev-T are connected by shaded bars.

sequences by <u>in situ</u> hybridization with <u>v-rel</u> probes and
with subclones of molecular clones of cellular DNA
obtained with <u>v-rel</u> probes.   Using a modification of the
method of Southern (Chen and Temin 1980), the authen-
ticity of the molecular clones as well as their relative
orientation was confirmed.   A restriction enzyme cleavage
map of an allele (see below) of <u>c-rel</u> from turkey 7 is
shown in Fig. 2.

RELATIONSHIP BETWEEN <u>c-rel</u> AND <u>v-rel</u>

     The regions of homology between <u>c-rel</u> (turkey 7) and
<u>rel</u> have been determined by restriction enzyme cleavage
site mapping and nucleic acid hybridization with <u>v-rel</u>
subclones.   The size and positions of some regions of
homology between <u>c-rel</u> and <u>v-rel</u> have been determined

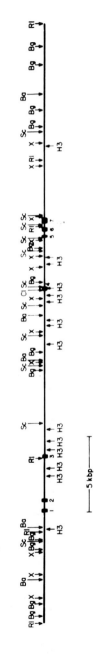

Fig. 2. Restriction Enzyme Cleavage Site Map of c-rel (turkey 7)

The restriction enzyme cleavage site map is a composite based on restriction enzyme cleavage site maps of molecular clones and genomic restriction enzyme cleavage site mapping. The regions of homology between v-rel and c-rel are shown as black boxes and are labeled 1 through 7. The size and position of regions 1, 2, and 3 are based on restriction enzyme cleavage site mapping, hence their exact size and position are not known. Regions 4, 5, 6, and 7 are positioned and their sizes based on measurement of 10 electron microscopic heteroduplexes. The termini of the molecular clones used are as follows: the 5' most Eco RI site to the Eco RI site 3' to region 2, the Eco RI site within region 3 to the Eco RI site 3' to region 6 and the Eco RI site 5' to region 7 to the 3' most Eco RI site shown.

more precisely by electron microscopic heteroduplex analysis of the c-rel (turkey 7) recombinant DNA clones and an REV-T provirus REV-T (Ch4A Rev-T 52B). There are seven regions of homology between v-rel and c-rel (turkey 7) spread over approximately 25 kbp. Electron microscopic heteroduplex analysis and nucleic acid hybridization data indicate that portions of v-rel are homologous to one and only one of the seven regions found in c-rel. The sizes of the regions of homology vary between 490 bp (region 7) to less than 100 bp (region 1).

The structural relationship between oncogenes and proto-oncogenes has been studied for other oncogenes (for examples see Oskarsson et al. 1980; Takeya et al. 1981; Ellis et al. 1981; Robins et al. 1982). Some oncogenes and proto-oncogenes are colinear with their oncogenes with only a few base changes (for example, c-mos, c-rasI). Other oncogenes have one or two segments of DNA interrupting the regions of homology between the respective proto-oncogene and oncogene (for example, c-myc, c-rasII). Other oncogenes have many segments of DNA, some of which are quite large, that interrupt the regions of homology in proto-oncogenes to their respective oncogenes (for example, c-src, c-erbB). c-rel is similar to the latter.

In many eukaryotic genes, sequences are present that interrupt the coding sequences of the gene (Jeffreys and Flavel 1977). These sequences, called introns, are spliced out of RNA transcripts prior to translation. It is believed that segments of DNA in proto-oncogenes that interrupt the sequences homologous to oncogenes are introns. Assuming the sequences in c-rel (turkey 7) that are not present in v-rel are introns explains the disparity between the approximately 25 kbp length of c-rel (turkey 7) and the 1.4 kbp length of v-rel. Shimotohno and Temin have been shown that if a cellular gene with introns is inserted in a spleen necrosis virus vector, the introns are lost during virus replication (Shimotohno and Temin 1982).

Recently, genes have been inserted into avian retroviruses vectors in vitro. It has been observed that modifications of these genes is necessary for their efficient transduction. These modifications are postulated to be general requirements for transduction of

all genes including proto-oncogenes. Shimotohno and
Temin determined that the 3' terminal sequences of the
mRNA of herpes sipmlex thymidine kinase needed to be
removed for its efficient propogation in a spleen
necrosis virus vector (Shimotohno and Temin 1981). If
the signal for the 3' terminus of an RNA transcript is
present 5' to the required 3' LTR of the retrovirus, a
functional virus will not be formed.

We found a 4 kb polyadenylated RNA transcript in
chicken cells (chicken c-rel will be later shown to be
closely related to turkey c-rel). This RNA is homologous
to v-rel, c-rel exons, and sequences 3' to the 3' most
exon (region 7) of c-rel, but it is not homologous
introns (Chen et al. 1982). This result indicates that
the 4 kb RNA cellular transcript of c-rel terminates 3'
to the sequences homologous to v-rel. The c-rel mRNA 3'
terminal sequences have not been transduced in Rev-T. In
each of the other proto-oncogenes for which a cellular
mRNA transcript has been found, the RNA transcripts are
at least 1 kb longer than their respective oncogene.
This size difference indicates that the loss of mRNA
terminal sequences is a general feature of the transduction of proto-oncogenes.

Since oncogenes in retroviruses give rise to tumors
and proto-oncogenes appear to be a normal non-tumorigenic
component of host genomic DNA, evidence for changes in
coding sequences is of interest. Since there are not
intervening sequences in v-rel, restriction enzme
cleavage sites found in v-rel should be present in the
corresponding regions of homology in c-rel. By sub-
cloning the v-rel sequences on either side of a restriction enzyme cleavage site and hybridizing each subclone
to c-rel, one can determine which exon should contain the
site found in v-rel. It is then a simple matter to
determine if there is an appropriate cleavage site in c-
rel.

There are two Eco RI cleavage sites in v-rel. One
is found in c-rel. The Eco RI site at 4.2 kbp in Rev-T
should be found in exon 7, but it is not present. Two
other restriction enzyme cleavage sites are also not
conserved (Bam HI at 3.25 kbp and Pst 1 at 4.4 kb of Rev-
T). Two sites have been conserved (Cla I at 4.55 kbp and
HindIII at 4.65 kpb of Rev-T).

The lack of conservation of a restriction enzyme cleavage site can not be assumed to correspond to an amino acid sequence change because of the degeneracy of the genetic code. Additionally, it can not be determined if the proto-oncogene studied is the allele from which an oncogene was transduced. A polymorphic allele of c-rel may exist which has identical coding sequences with v-rel. The difference between such an allele and the alle in turkey 7 would then have been generated either by somatic mutation and/or evolutionary divergence of germ line sequences.

POLYMORPHISM IN c-rel(turkey)

To determine the incidence and nature of polymorphism in c-rel, a small collection of unrelated turkey embryos were examined (Fig. 3). The DNAs were cleaved with Eco RI, electrophoresed in an agarose gel, transferred to nitrocellulose, and hybridized to v-rel-containing probes. The probes used in this study were three subclones of Rev-T that divide v-rel into three nonoverlapping regions. The junction between these subclones are the Eco RI sites at 3.5 and 4.2 kbp. For each of the embryos analyzed, a 1.0 kb EcoRI fragment was detected that hybridized both to the 5' and middle v-rel probes. Similarly a 4.4 kb EcoRI fragment from each of the embryos hybridized to both the middle and 3' v-rel probes. These results allow us to show that the Eco RI site at 4.2 kbp in Rev-T is not conserved in these four embryos. [The 1.0 kbp EcoRI fragment appears to be a duplication of part of c-rel (unpublished data).]

Each of the embryos analyzed (Fig. 3) has one or two large EcoRI fragments which hybridize to the middle v-rel probe. The simplest model to explain this observation is that there is one locus for c-rel with at least two possible alleles. Molecular clones have been obtained of two allelic EcoRI fragments from an apparently hetero-zygous turkey embryo. Electron microscopic heteroduplex analysis of these two clones shows that they differ by a substitution. The larger EcoRI fragment contains 2.4 kb not present in the smaller EcoRI fragment. While the smaller EcoRI fragment contains 0.17 kb not found in the larger EcoRI fragment. This substitution is in an intron just 5' to exon 4 (Fig. 2).

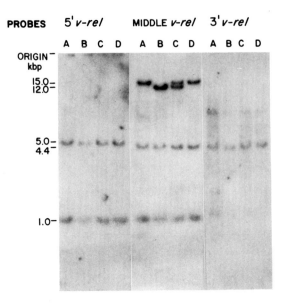

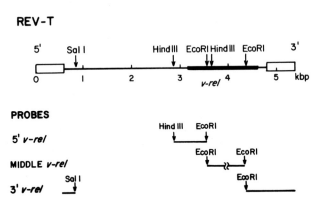

Fig. 3. Polymorphism of c-rel in Turkey
DNA from four unrelated turkey embryos, A, B, C and D (A, B, and C are Orlopp turkeys; D is a Bronze turkey; C is from embryo 7) was digested with Eco RI, electrophoresed on a 0.5% agarose gel, transferred to nitrocellulose and hybridized with either 5', middle or 3' v-rel probes (see text). A restriction enzyme cleavage site map of Rev-T DNA and subcloned fragments used to make 5', middle and 3' v-rel probes are shown below.

In addition to the substitution detected in c-rel alleles, we found another form of polymorphism. Molecular clones from two embryos were obtained which contain exon number 7 and 3' flanking sequences. Restriction enzyme cleavage maps of molecular clones from this region are shown in Fig. 4. Close to exon 7 both molecular clones have identical restriction enzyme cleavage sites patterns. Further 3', however, there is an increased incidence of discordant restriction enzyme cleavage sites. Electron microscopic heteroduplex analysis and filter hybridization, which are insensitive to small amounts of mismatching, indicate that the 3' flanking regions are homologous overall. Therefore, the observed restriction enzyme cleavage site differences are the result of base changes.

COMPARISON OF c-rel(turkey) AND c-rel(chicken)

In addition to our studies of turkey DNA, we molecularly cloned c-rel from a chicken embryo in a manner similar to that used for c-rel from turkey (Chen et al. 1982). Fig. 5 shows a restriction enzyme cleavage site map and the regions of homology between v-rel and chicken DNA. The size and number of exons is conserved in c-rel chicken and turkey. There are, however, many restriction enzyme cleavage site differences in introns, as would be expected. Exons 1 and 2, are separated by different amounts in chicken and turkey.

Electron microscopic heteroduplex analysis between chicken and turkey clones demonstrated that between exons 3 and 4 there are two unequal length substitutions in the intervening sequence. Similarly, between exons 4 and 5 and within 5 kbp of exon 7, there is also an unequal length substitution. Greater than 5 kbp 3' to exon 7 chicken and turkey are not homologous. Areas in introns were also detected where mismatching in regions of homology caused heteroduplexes to denature frequently. A composite diagram of a comparison of c-rel from chicken and turkey is shown in Fig. 6.

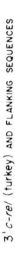
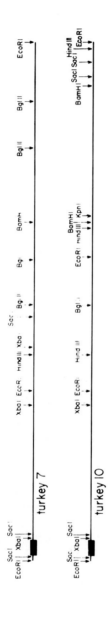

Fig. 4. Polymorphism of 3' c-rel Flanking Sequence

Restriction enzyme cleavage site maps for the inserts of molecular clones from the 3' end of c-rel from turkey embryos 7 and 10 are diagrammed. The region of homology between c-rel and v-rel is drawn as a bar and corresponds to region 7 in Fig. 2.

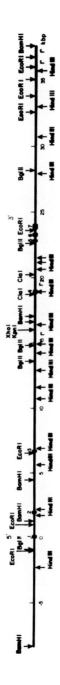

Fig. 5. c-rel (chicken)

The restriction enzyme cleavage site map of c-rel (chicken) is based on four over-lapping molecular clones that were obtained from recombinate DNA libraries prepared from DNA of a single individual (from flock 15B) (Chen et al. 1983). The regions of homology between v-rel and c-rel (chicken) are shown as boxes and labeled 1 through 7. Regions 1 through 7 were positioned by restriction enzyme cleavage site mapping and hybridization. The size and positions of regions 4, 5, 6 and 7 are equivalent to those in turkey and are drawn accordingly.

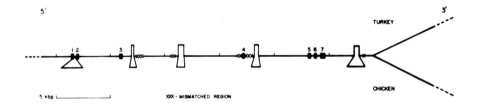

Fig. 6. Differences between c-rel Chicken and Turkey

Regions of homology between chicken and turkey are drawn as single line. Regions of homology between chicken and turkey in which there is a high frequency of mis-matches are marked X. Regions with no homology are shown with lines above the center line for turkey and below the center line for chicken. The regions of homology between v-rel and c-rel are shown as boxes and numbered as in Figures 2 and 4. There are different lengths in chickens and turkey between regions 1 and 2 or between regions 2 and 3. These unequal lengths are assumed to be the result of insertions. 3' to region 3, the map is based on electron microscopic heteroduplex analysis of molecular clones of chicken and turkey. The turkey clone allele that was used in this study is the larger of the two shown in Figure 2. The substitutions between regions 3 and 6 are drawn such that the larger strand of the susbstitution is present in chickens. This decision was based on the lengths of the distance between regions 3 and 6 in chicken and turkey. The substitution 3' to region 7 could be longer in turkey or in chicken.

SUMMARY

The process of transduction of a proto-oncogene involves the loss of intervening sequences, the loss of 3' mRNA terminal sequences, and possible base changes. It is not possible to know how similar the c-rel sequences we studied are to sequences from which v-rel arose. If one of the alleles we studied is identical to progenitor sequences of v-rel, then base changes must have occurred during the process of transduction. Alternatively, there may exist an allele of c-rel which did not need to undergo base changes to give rise to v-rel.

The polymorphism of c-rel within a turkey population and between chicken and turkey shows clear evidence of base changes within noncoding regions. Polymorphism in c-rel coding sequences have not been detected within a turkey population. There is an EcoRI site in c-rel from turkey which is not in v-rel. There are unequal length substitutions in c-rel within the turkey population and between chicken and turkey. Unequal length substitutions can be explained if there has been a combination of two events, for example, insertion or deletion with extensive base changes, or two insertions or deletions. Two events occurring in a short evolutionary time span might occur if c-rel is diverging at a relatively fast rate. c-rel is much less conserved across species lines, in nucleic acid hybridization to v-rel (Chen et al. 1981; Wong and Lai 1981) than other proto-oncogenes, consistent with it diverging at a relatively fast rate.

Since the evolutionary changes that have been seen for c-rel are in noncoding sequences, it is most likely that v-rel arose by transduction of a somatic mutation generated variant of c-rel or by transduction which involves sequence changes or later mutations.

Bishop JM, Varmus H (1982) Functions and origins of retroviral oncogenes. In Weiss R, Teich N, Varmus HE Coffin J (eds): "Molecular Biology of Tumor Viruses: RNA Tumor Viruses," New York: Cold Spring Harbor.

Blattner FR, Williams BG, Blechl AE, Denniston-Thompson K, Faber HE, Furlong LA, Grunwald DJ, Keifer DO, Moore DO, Schumn JW, Sheldon EI, Smithies O (1977) Charon phages: safer derivatives of bacteriophage lambda for DNA cloning. Science 196:161.

Breitman ML, Lai MMC, Vogt PK (1980) The genomic RNA of avian reticuloendotheliosis virus REV. Virology 100:50.

Chen ISY, Temin HM (1980) Ribonucleotides in unintegrated linear spleen necrosis virus. J Virol 33:1058.

Chen ISY, Mak TW, O'Rear JJ, Temin HM (1981) Characterization of reticuloendotheliosis virus strain T DNA and isolation of a novel variant of reticuloendotheliosis virus strain T by molecular cloning. J Virol 40:800.

Chen ISY, Wilhelmsen KC, Temin HM (1983) The structure of c-rel the cellular homologue of the oncogene Rev-T. J Virol in press.

Ellis RW, Defoe D, Shih TY, Gonda MA, Young MA, Tsuchida N, Lowy DR, Scolnick EM (1981) The p21 src genes of Harvey and Kirsten sarcoma viruses originate from divergent members of family of normal vertebrate genes. Science 292:506.

Gonda MA, Rice NR, Gilden RV (1980) Avian reticuloendotheliosis virus: Characterization of high-molecular-weight viral RNA in transforming and helper virus populations. J Virol 34:743.

Hu SSF, Lai MMC, Wang TC, Cohen RS, Sovian M (1981) Avian reticuloendotheliosis virus: Characterization of genomic structure by heteroduplex mapping. J Virol 37:899.

Jeffreys AJ, Flavell RA (1977) The rabbin β globin gene contains a large insert in the coding sequence. Cell 12:1097.

Karn J, Brenner S, Barnett L, Cesareni G (1980) Novel bacteriophage λ cloning vector. PNAS 77:5172.

Oskarsson M, Mclements WL, Blair DG, Maizel JV, Van de Woude GF (1980) Properties of a normal mouse cell DNA sequence (sarc) homologous to the src sequence of Moloney sarcoma virus. Science 207:1222.

Robins T, Blister K, Garon C, Papas T, Duesberg P (1982) Structural relationship between a normal chicken DNA locus and the transforming gene of the avian acute leukemia virus MC29. J Virol 41:635.

Shimotohno K, Temin HM (1981) Formation of infectious progeny virus after insertion of herpes thymidine kinase gene into DNA of an avian retrovirus. Cell 26:67.

Shimotohno K, Temin HM (1982) Loss of intervening sequences in genomic mouse α-globin DNA inserted in an infectious retrovirus vector. Nature in press.

Takeya T, Hanafusa M, Junghans RP, JU G, Skalka AM (1981) Comparison between the viral tranfsorming gene (src) of recovered avian sarcoma virus and its cellular homology. Mol Cell Biol 1:1024.

Thelien GH, Zeigel RF, Twiehaus MJ (1966) Biological studies with RE virus (strain T) that induces reticulo-endotheliosis in turkeys, chicken, and Japanese quail.

Wong TC, Lai MMC (1981) Avian reticuloendotheliosis virus contains a new class of oncogene of turkey origin. Virol 111:289.

Oncogenes and Retroviruses: Evaluation of Basic Findings and Clinical Potential, pages 57–63
© **1983 Alan R. Liss, Inc., 150 Fifth Avenue, New York, NY 10011**

STRUCTURE AND FUNCTION OF THE ABELSON MURINE LEUKEMIA VIRUS
TRANSFORMING GENE

Jean Yin Jen Wang, Ron Prywes and David Baltimore
Whitehead Institute for Biomedical Research
Massachusetts Institute of Technology
Cambridge, Massachusetts 02139

INTRODUCTION

Abelson murine leukemia virus (A-MuLV) was isolated from
a lymphoma which was induced by infection of a steroid-treated
mouse with Moloney-MuLV (M-MuLV) (Abelson and Rabstein, 1970).
It has been established that A-MuLV is a derivative of M-MuLV
(Shields et al., 1979) but, unlike M-MuLV, A-MuLV induces a
lymphoma of the B lymphocyte lineage and it can transform
these and fibroblastic cells in vitro (Rosenberg and Baltimore,
1976; Scher and Siegler, 1975). A-MuLV has a hybrid genome
as shown in Fig. 1. It contains M-MuLV sequences on the 5'-
and 3'-ends but has a stretch of unique sequence, v-abl, in
the middle. A-MuLV encodes one protein of 160,000 molecular
weight which initiates in the M-MuLV gag sequences and reads
through and terminates within v-abl (Witte et al., 1978).

Relationship between v-abl and c-abl

The v-abl sequence is derived from the mouse genome and
evidence of homologous sequence in vertebrate genomes has
been obtained (Goff et al., 1980). To analyze the relationship between v-abl and the homologous cellular sequences
(c-abl), a v-abl probe was constructed and used to isolate
c-abl sequences on λ bacteriophage vectors. Although v-abl
is only 4.3 kb, c-abl sequences were found to be distributed
along 30 kb of mouse DNA (Fig. 2). When the cloned DNA was
digested with restriction enzymes and probed with different
sections of the v-abl sequence, the locations of c-abl were

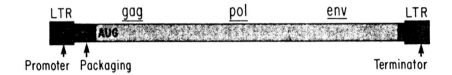

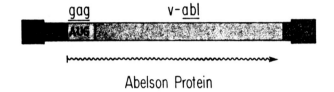

Abelson Protein

Fig. 1 Structure of A-MuLV

identified and the correlation between v-abl and c-abl could be made (Fig. 2). The 3'-half of the v-abl is colinear with 2 kb of the mouse DNA, but the 5'-half of the v-abl is divided into at least eight small sections spanning 20 kb of the cloned DNA.

The distribution of c-abl sequences resembles that of a normal cellular split gene. The RNA transcripts of this gene were identified by hybridization with v-abl probes and two species of 6.5 kb and 5.5 kb were found in various mouse tissues and cell lines (Wang and Baltimore, in preparation). The v-abl sequence can be related to the two c-abl RNA as shown in Fig. 3. We found that the v-abl sequence is colinear with the c-abl RNA but represents only the internal sequence of the c-abl transcripts.

By comparing the nucleotide sequences of M-MuLV, c-abl and A-MuLV, the junctions between M-MuLV and v-abl on both 5'- and 3'-ends were defined. Interestingly, we found a

four-base pair homology between M—MuLV and c-abl at the 5'
junction. Because short homologies in DNA are known to
catalyze recombination or deletion events, it is likely that

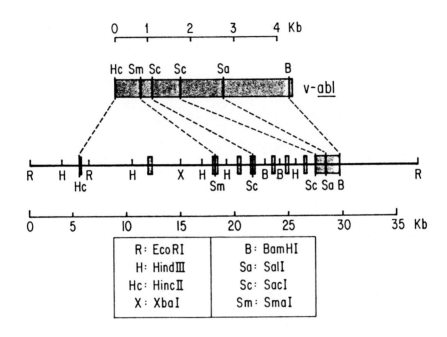

Fig. 2 Relationship between v-abl and c-abl

the 5' junction of A-MuLV was formed at DNA level by interaction between an integrated M—MuLV genome and c-abl. As
shown in Fig. 4, this deletion fusion event would result in
the transcription of a hybrid RNA from the M—MuLV LTR promoter.
This precursor hybrid RNA could then recombine with a M—MuLV
RNA to generate the A-MuLV RNA genome.

v-abl Encodes a Tyrosine Kinase

The hybrid protein of A-MuLV was shown to become phosphorylated on tyrosine residues in an immunoprecipitated form
(Witte et al., 1980a). The A-MuLV protein was shown to be a
tyrosine-specific protein kinase by expressing the v-abl coding

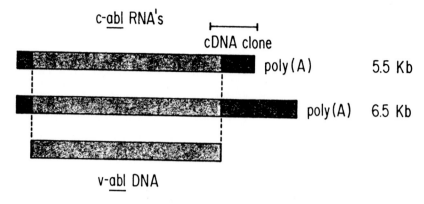

Fig. 3 Relationship between v-abl and c-abl RNA

sequence in E. coli. Bacteria containing the v-abl encoded protein had tyrosine-phosphorylated proteins whereas normal E. coli contained no detectable amount of phosphotyrosine (Wang et al., 1982). Only 1.2 kb of the 5'-end of the v-abl sequence was sufficient to code for the tyrosine kinase. The M-MuLV gag sequences are not necessary for the coding of protein kinase activity. The v-abl encoded protein can phosphorylate itself as well as bacterial proteins on tyrosine residues.

The Minimal Transforming Region of the A-MuLV Genome

The genomes of two naturally occurring variants of A-MuLV have been cloned (Goff et al., 1980; Latt et al., 1982). The A-MuLV(P160) genome is colinear with the c-abl RNA whereas the A-MuLV(P120) genome has an internal deletion of 800 bp (Fig. 5). Because both viruses transform cells with equal efficiency, the deleted sequence must not be necessary for transformation. An early termination mutant of A-MuLV(P120) gives rise to a P90 protein capable of transformation, thus sequences beyond the end of P90 are also dispensable. The dispensability of these sequences is further demonstrated by introducing a premature termination in the A-MuLV(P160) genome within the naturally occurred deletion region of A-MuLV(P120). This virus produces a protein of 105,000 molecular weight and it transforms both fibroblasts and pre-B cells.

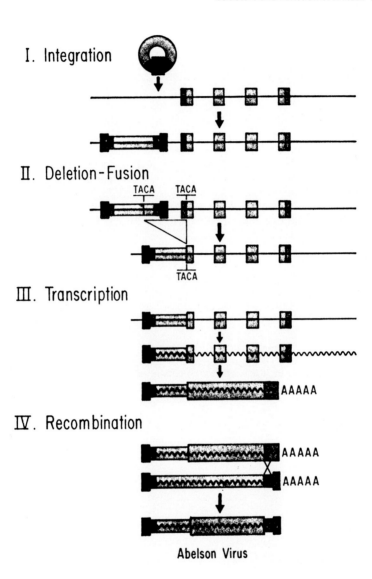

I. Integration

II. Deletion-Fusion

III. Transcription

IV. Recombination

Abelson Virus

Fig. 4 Model for the formation of A-MuLV

As described before, the M-MuLV <u>gag</u> sequences are not
needed for the production of an active tyrosine kinase. The
elimination of all but 100 base pairs of the <u>gag</u> coding region
also generated a transforming virus. Therefore, 90% of the
<u>gag</u> region can be removed from A-MuLV without any effect on
the transformation of fibroblasts. The 5'-break point of the
A-MuLV(P120) deletion is 20 base pairs from a PstI site. A
minimal transforming virus was made by removing all the v-<u>abl</u>
sequences 3' to that PstI site from the A-MuLV-<u>gag</u>⁻ genome
(Fig. 5). This virus produced a 52,000 molecular weight protein which induced the transformation of fibroblasts. Apparently, the A-MuLV genome can be trimmed down substantially
without affecting its ability to transform fibroblasts. The
5'-1.2 kb v-<u>abl</u> region is necessary because a mutant with a
700 bp deletion in this region is transformation defective
(Witte et al., 1980b).

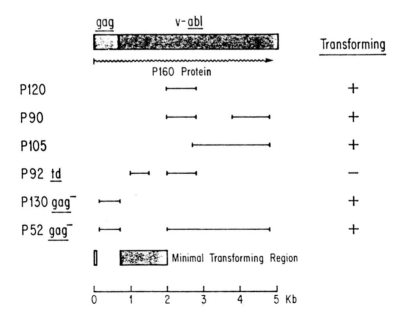

Fig. 5 Definition of the minimal transforming region of A-MuLV
⊢————⊣ represents deletions.

Summary

The oncogene (v-abl) of A-MuLV is a fragment of a normal mouse gene. Only 1.2 kb on the 5'-end of the v-abl is sufficient to encode a tyrosine-specific protein kinase whose activity is important in transformation. This A-MuLV protein kinase can be active in E. coli and it phosphorylates bacterial proteins. The lack of discrimination in its selection for substrates is puzzling. Because of the demonstration of such promiscuity, the identification of physiologically-relevant phosphorylation events must rely on evidence of functional modification rather than physical modification of proteins.

Abelson HT, Rabstein LS (1970). Influence of prednisolone on Moloney leukemia virus in BALB/c mice. Cancer Res 30:2208-2212.

Goff SP, Gilboa E, Witte ON, Baltimore, D (1980). Structure of the Abelson murine leukemia virus genome and the homologous cellular gene: studies with cloned viral DNA. Cell 22:777-785.

Latt S, Goff SP, Tabin C, Paskind M, Wang JYJ, Baltimore D (1982). Cloning and analysis of reverse transcript (P160) genomes of Abelson murine leukemia virus. J Virol submitted.

Rosenberg N, Baltimore D (1976). A quantitative assay for transformation of bone marrow cells by Abelson murine leukemia virus. J Exp Med 143:1453-1463.

Scher CD, Siegler R (1975). Direct transformation of 3T3 cells by Abelson murine leukemia virus. Nature (Lond) 253:729-732.

Shields A, Goff SP, Paskind M, Otto G, Baltimore D (1979). Structure of the Abelson murine leukemia virus genome. Cell 18:955-962.

Wang JYJ, Baltimore D (1982). RNA transcripts of the cellular homologue of the Abelson viral transforming gene: expression and relationship with the viral sequence, in preparation.

Wang JYJ, Queen C, Baltimore D (1982). Expression of Abelson murine leukemia virus genome causes extensive tyrosine-phosphorylation in E. coli. J Biol Chem, in press.

Witte ON, Dasgupta A, Baltimore D (1980a). Abelson murine leukemia virus protein is phosphorylated in vitro to form phosphotyrosine. Nature 283:826-831.

Witte ON, Goff S, Rosenberg N, Baltimore D (1980b). A transformation-defective mutant of Abelson murine leukemia virus lacks protein kinase activity. Proc Natl Acad Sci USA 77:4993-4997.

Witte ON, Rosenberg N, Paskind M, Shields A, Baltimore D (1978). Identification of an Abelson murine leukemia virus-encoded protein present in transformed fibroblasts and lymphoid cells. Proc Natl Acad Sci USA 75:2488-2492.

TRANSFECTION STUDIES

Oncogenes and Retroviruses: Evaluation of Basic Findings
and Clinical Potential, pages 67–77
© 1983 Alan R. Liss, Inc., 150 Fifth Avenue, New York, NY 10011

EXPRESSION OF ENDOGENOUS p21 ras GENES

Ronald W. Ellis, Deborah DeFeo, Alex Papageorge,
and Edward M. Scolnick
Virus and Cell Biology Research
Merck Sharp & Dohme Research Laboratories
West Point, PA 19486

Our laboratory has been studying the molecular biology
of the ras oncogene family, which encodes a set of 21,000
dalton transforming proteins called p21 ras (Ellis et. al.,
1982). This family is divisible into two groups (Ellis
et. al., 1981), based upon the relationship to the Harvey
(Ha) or Kirsten (Ki) strains of murine sarcoma virus (MuSV);
The p21 ras polypeptides encoded by these two viruses cross-
react serologically (Shih et al., 1979) and share 85% of
their amino acids (Dhar et al., 1982; Tsuchida et al., 1982).
Nevertheless, their nucleotide coding sequences have accumulated so many changes in the third base codon position
that cloned DNA probes from each viral (v) ras gene cross-
hybridize poorly under stringent conditions (Ellis et al.,
1981). This relative lack of crossreactivity has been
exploited to detect distinct sets of cellular (c) Ha ras
and Ki ras sequences in a range of vertebrate species (Ellis
et al., 1980, 1981), several of which have been cloned (De-
Feo et al., 1981; Chang et al., 1982).

As an approach toward understanding the function of
cellular p21 ras, we have been studying the expression of
ras genes in non-malignant cells. 416B mouse cells, which
share some biological properties with early hemopoietic
stem cells (Dexter et al, 1979). are useful for this purpose,
in that their markedly elevated levels (compared to normal
cells, see Scolnick et al., 1981) of p21 facilitate studies
of c ras gene expression, of the number of mRNAs potentially encoding p21, and of c ras p21 itself.

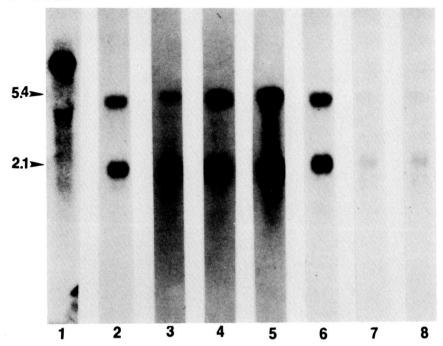

Figure 1.   Northern blot analysis with Ki ras-specific
probe.   Cellular RNAs were electrophoresed, blotted, and
hybridized to ^{32}P -labeled Ki ras DNA (Ellis et al.,
1981), as described elsewhere (Ellis et al, 1982).   Lane 1,
Ki-NIH total cellular RNA; Lane 2, 416B total cellular RNA;
Lane 3, 416B nuclear RNA; Lane 4, 416B cytoplasmic RNA;
Lane 5, 416B poly A+ RNA; Lane 6, 416B polysomal RNA; Lane
7, 427E total cellular RNA; Lane 8, NIH total cellular RNA.
The lengths of the RNAs (in Kb) were judged relative to 28S
and 18S ribosomal RNA markers.

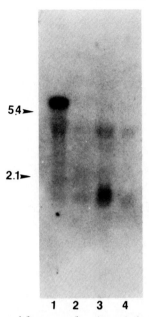

54►

2.1►

1 2 3 4

Figure 2. Northern blot analysis with Ha ras-specific
probe. Cellular RNAs were electrophoresed, blotted, and
hybridized to ^{32}P Ha ras DNA (Ellis et al., 1980). Total
cellular RNA preparations were from: Lane 1, Ha-NIH; Lane
2, 416B; Lane 3, 427E; Lane 4, NIH.

      Our group has utilized monoclonal antibodies against
p21 ras to study protein expression in transformed and
normal cells (Furth et al., 1982). The use of antibodies
which can discriminate between Ha or Ki p21 ras has
suggested that the predominant p21 ras expressed in 416B
cells is Ki-related. Therefore, to begin to understand
the molecular basis for p21 ras amplification in 416B
cells, we studied the expression of Ki ras cellular RNA
by the Northern blotting technique. RNA preparations
from 416B, 427E (a cell line originating from the same
F-MuLV-infected BDF$_1$ bone marrow culture as 416B and
containing normal levels of c ras p21), Ki-MuSV-infected
NIH 3T3 (K-NIH), and NIH 3T3 (NIH) cells were electrophoresed, blotted, and hybridized to a Ki ras-specific probe
(Figure 1). It is clear that 416B, 427E, and NIH cells
contain two Ki ras-related RNA species sized 5.2 and 2.0
kb and indistinguishable in size among the cell lines
(lanes 2,7,8). By means of variable exposure times of the

autoradiograph, we estimate that 416B cells contain
approximately 25-fold more Ki ras RNA than do the other
mouse cells.

In order to confirm that the high levels of p21 expressed in 416B cells are Ki ras-rather than Ha ras-related
RNA preparations from 416B, 427E, Ha-MuSV-infected NIH
(Ha-NIH), and NIH cells were electrophoresed, blotted,
and hybridized to a Ha ras specific probe (Figure 2).
These cell lines all contained two Ha ras-related RNA
species which were smaller than Ha-MuSV mRNA (lane 1) and
whose sizes (5.0 and 1.4 kb) were distinct from the two Ki
ras-related RNAs, as determined by mixing experiments (data
not shown). Notably, the levels of these RNAs in 416B cells
were not substantially different from those in the other
cell lines. Since it has been reported that 416B cells are
not infected with the Ha-MuSV, Ki-MuSV, or any other agent
potentially encoding p21 (Scolnick et al., 1981), these
results confirm that the high levels of p21 ras in this
cell line originate from an endogenous c Ki ras gene
rather than an endogenous c Ha ras gene.

Having established the Ki ras origin of the amplified
416B p21, evidence then was sought for a possible processing or functional relationship between these two RNA species
in 416B cells. Both unselected and poly A-selected 416B
cellular RNA contained the 5.2 and 2.0 kb species in
approximately equimolar ratios (Figure 1, lanes 2 and 5),
suggesting that both contain poly A. Both molecules
appeared to be polysome-associated, as judged by EDTA release from purified polyribosomes (lane 6). Finally, both
nuclear and cytoplasmic RNA preparations contained the two
species in similar molar ratios (lanes 4 and 5), suggesting
that the two share no clear precursor/product relationship.
In summary, 416B cells contain two Ki ras related RNA species which are independent, poly A+, and polyribosome-associ-
ated and whose expression is amplified approximately 25-
fold over levels of similarly-sized RNAs in other mouse
cell lines.

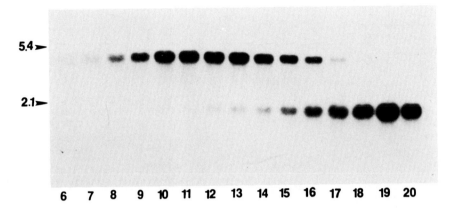

Figure 3. Northern blot analysis with Ki ras-specific probe. 416B total cellular RNA was isolated and resolved on a continuous 10-40% sucrose density gradient as described (Ellis et al., 1982). Aliquots of individual gradient fractions, as numbered, were electrophoresed, blotted, and hybridized to ^{32}P labeled Ki ras DNA.

   The data presented in Figure 1 suggest that both the 5.2 and the 2.0 kb RNA molecules are capable of functioning as mRNAs encoding c Ki ras p21. In 416B cells the abundance of these RNAs enables us to test this possibility directly. Total 416B cellular RNA was centrifuged through a 10-40% continuous sucrose density gradient. Individual fractions were tested for the presence of the 5.2 and 2.0 kbp RNAs by gel electrophoresis, blotting, and hybridization with a Ki ras probe. Figure 3 demonstrates our ability to resolve these two species; in particular, note the relative underrepresentation of each band in fractions 16-17 as compared to the peaks in fractions 10-13 (5.2 kb) and fractions 19-20 (2.0 kb). An aliquot of each fraction was used to prime a nuclease-digested rabbit reticulocyte lysate for in vitro translation. Proteins translated in vitro were immunoprecipitated with a monoclonal antibody against p21, electrophoresed, and the gels were autoradiographed, as shown in Figure 4. Fractions from both RNA hybridization peaks (Figure 6, 10-13 and 19-20) stimulated the synthesis of the greatest amount of p21, while intermediate fractions (16-18) primed substantially less synthesis. Fraction 2 (panel A), which

contains very little c Ki ras RNA detected by Northern
blotting, stimulates little p21 synthesis above the background of the zero RNA control (lane 0). The difference
in migration between p21 molecules prepared by in vitro
translation and by ^{35}S-methionine labelling (panel B,
lanes 2 and 4) may reflect the lack of protein processing
in vitro which does occur in the intact cells (Shih et al.,
1982). Even though the correlation for individual fractions between mRNA levels and stimulation of p21 synthesis
was not an absolute one, both the 5.2 kb peak fractions and
the 2.0 kb peak fractions primed synthesis of p21 polypeptides which were indistinguishable in size by polyacrylamide gel electrophoresis. These data demonstrate that
both the 5.2 and the 2.0 kb RNAs can function as mRNAs for
c Ki ras p21.

Our results have demonstrated that mouse cells contain
two RNA species homologous to Ha ras and two homologous to
Ki ras. In the case of the Ki ras mRNAs in 416B cells, we
find that both mRNA species can be translated in vitro
into p21; these mRNAs are indistinguishable in size from
those in other mouse cells. These data suggest that mouse
cells contain two mRNAs which encode Ki ras p21 and, by
analogy, two which encode Ha ras p21. The presence of
more than one cellular mRNA encoding a specific onc protein
may be a fairly widespread phenomenon. Our description of
two distinct mRNA species able to be translated in vitro
into p21 ras represents the first description of such a
phenomenon for any individual cellular onc protein.

The coding sequences for both Ha ras and Ki ras p21
are approximately 0.65 kb in length (Dhar et al., 1982,
Tsuchida et al, 1982). This means that the 4 ras mRNAs in
mouse cells, being sized over a range of 1.4-5.4 kb, contain two-to eight-fold as much coding capacity as is
necessary for their translated proteins. It is interesting
to consider the disposition of the ras coding sequences
relative to the 5' and 3' ends of these mRNAs. Data from
other genetic systems suggest that the amount of untranslated RNA at the 3' end of mRNAs can be variable (Heilig
et al., 1980, Setzer et al., 1980), implying that the
difference between the two Ki ras mRNAs in 416B might lie
in the length of their respective 3' untranslated sequences.
The function of this putatively extra RNA is unknown. It
is interesting to speculate whether the extra nucleotide
sequences are important in the regulation of expression of
these mRNAs.

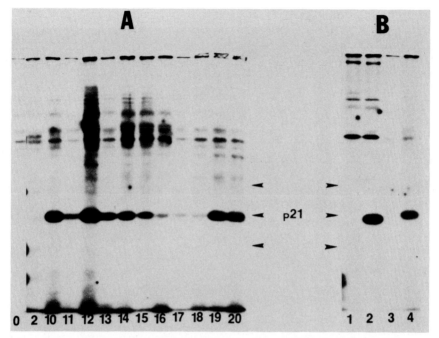

Figure 4. Gel electrophoresis of immunoprecipitates from
in vitro translations. Panel A. Aliquots of fractions
from the sucrose density gradient of Figure 3 were used to
prime in vitro translation in a rabbit reticulocyte lysate,
utilizing ^{35}S methionine. Immunoprecipitations were performed with the v ras monoclonal antibody 259, which immunoprecipitates both Ki ras and Ha ras p21 molecules (Furth et
al., 1982). Lane 0, RNA control; Lanes 10-20, portions of
fractions 10-20 of Figure 3 used for priming in vitro translation. Panel B. Lanes 1,2. 416B cells were labeled for
4h at 37°, and cell extracts were made as described (Shih
et al., 1979). Lanes 3,4. Gradient fraction 12 (Figure 3)
was used to prime in vitro translation, as described above.
Immunoprecipitations were performed with monoclonal antibody 259 (lanes 2,4) or the Ha ras-specific monoclonal antibody 172 (lanes 1,3). The arrows indicate molecular weight
markers: α-chymotrypsinogen (27,500) and β-lactoglobulin
(18,400).

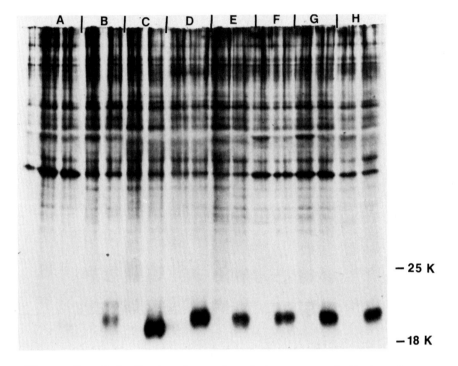

Figure 5. Gel electrophoresis of immunoprecipitates from
infected and transfected NIH 3T3 lines. Cell extracts
were prepared following in vivo labeling with ^{35}S methionine. The first lane in each pair is an immunoprecipitation
with control serum, the second lane with Ha-MuSV-specific
antiserum. A. Uninfected NIH 3T3 cells. B. NIH 3T3 cells
infected. C-**D.** NIH 3T3 transformants induced by transfection with the following DNA preparations: C. The viral
LTR ligated to human c Ha ras 1. D. EJ bladder carcinoma
oncogene. The arrows indicate molecular weight markers:
α-chymotrypsinogen (25,700) and β-lactoglobulin (18,400).

Recent reports have suggested a possible role for Ha
ras p21 and **Ki** ras p21 in human neoplasia. High molecular
weight cellular DNAs from certain human tumor cell lines
have been able to induce transformed cell foci in transfection assays, suggesting the presence of an active oncogene in the lines. Recently, the bladder transforming gene
(EJ) has been identified as human c Ha ras 1, and the

colon/lung transforming gene as human c **Ki** ras 1 (Parada et
al.,1982, Dhar et al., 1982, M. Barbacid, personal communication, M. Goldfarb and M. Wigler, personal communication).
Since the normal human c Ha ras 1 gene is incapable of inducing transformed cell foci without being ligated to retroviral LTR sequences (Chang et al., 1982), these results
suggest that there has been a qualitative or quantitative
change in p21 ras gene expression in these tumor lines.
In order to understand the nature of this change, we chose
to compare the p21 ras species expressed in NIH 3T3 cells
transformed by either human c Ha ras 1 (ligated to the LTR
sequences) or by the EJ bladder gene (Figure 5). Lane C
demonstrates that the p21 encoded by the normal human gene
migrates more rapidly than viral p21 ras (lane B). In
contrast, EJ bladder p21 ras (lane D) migrates more slowly
than normal human p21 ras. This strongly suggests that at
minimum, a qualitative change (i.e., a change in the coding
sequence) has occured in normal human c Ha ras 1 which has
rendered the gene capable of inducing cellular transformation.

   While it is important to keep in mind that the human
oncogenes characterized to this point are assayed by their
ability to induce foci in transfections of NIH 3T3 cells,
these genes may play a role in human neoplasia. Several
cellular oncogenes are transcribed in various human tumor
cells (Eva et al., 1982). Continued study of these genes,
particular Ha ras and Ki ras, by DNA sequence analysis and
by Northern blot analysis of expressed RNAs may shed light
on their biological roles.

References

Chang, E.H., Furth, M.E., Scolnick, E.M. and Lowy, D.R.,
   1982. Immunogenic transformation of mammalian cells
   induced by a normal human gene homologous to the oncogene
   of Harvey murine sarcoma virus. Nature 297, 479-483.
Chang, E.H., Gonda, M.A., Ellis, R.W., Scolnick, E.M. and
   Lowy, D.R., 1982. The human genome contains four genes
   homologous to the transforming genes of Harvey and Kirsten
   murine sarcoma viruses. Proc. Natl. Acad. Sci. U.S.A.
   79: 4848-4852.
DeFeo, D., Gonda, M.A., Young, H.A., Chang, E.H., Lowy, D.R.,
   Scolnick, E.M. and Ellis, R.W., 1981. Analysis of two
   divergent rat genomic clones homologous to the transforming gene of Harvey sarcoma virus. Proc. Natl. Acad. Sci.
   U.S.A. 78: 3328-3332.

Der, C.J., Krontiris, T.A. and Cooper, G.M., 1982. Transforming genes of human bladder and lung carcinoma cell
lines are homologous to the ras genes of Harvey and Kirsten sarcoma viruses. Proc. Natl. Acad. Sci. U.S.A. 79:
3637-3640.
Dexter, T.M., Allen, T.D., Scott, D., and Teich, N.M., 1979.
Isolation and characterization of a bipotential haematopoietic cell line. Nature (London) 277: 471-474.
Dhar, R., Ellis, R.W., Shih, T.Y., Oroszlan, S., Shapiro,
B., Maizel, J., Lowy, D., and Scolnick, E.M., 1982. The
nucleotide sequence of the p21 transforming protein of
Harvey murine sarcoma virus. Science: 217: 946-948.
Ellis, R.W., DeFeo, D., Maryak, J.M., Young, H.A., Shih, T.
Y., Chang, E.H., Lowy, D.R., Scolnick, E.M., 1980. Dual
evolutionary origin for the rat genetic sequences of Har-
vey murine sarcoma virus. J. Virology 36: 408-420.
Ellis, R.W., DeFeo, D., Shih, T.Y., Gonda, M.A., Young, H.A.,
Tsuchida, N., Lowy, D.R. and Scolnick, E.M., 1981. The
p21 src genes of Harvey and Kirsten murine sarcoma viruses
originate from divergent members of a family of normal
vertebrate genes. Nature (London) 292: 506-511.
Ellis, R.W., DeFeo, D., Furth,M. and Scolnick E.M., 1982.
Mouse cells contain two distinct ras gene messenger RNA
species which can be translated into a p21 onc protein.
Molecular and Cellular Biology. In press.
Ellis, R.W., Lowy, D.R., Scolnick, E.M., 1982. The viral
and cellular p21 (ras) gene family. In: Advances in
Viral Oncology (Volume 1): Cell-derived Oncogenes, edited
by G. Klein, 107-126, Raven Press, New York.
Eva, A., Robbins, K.C., Andersen, P.R., Srinivasan, A.,
Tronick, S.R., Premkumar Reddy, E., Ellmore, N.W., Galen,
A.T., Lautenberger, J.A., Papas, T.S., Westin, E.H., Wong-
Staal, F., Gallo, R.C. and Aaronson, S.A., 1982. Cellu-
lar genes analogous to retroviral onc genes are transcribed
in human tumor cells. Nature (London) 295: 116-119.
Furth, M.E., Davis, L.J., Fleurdelys, B., Scolnick, E.M.,
1982. Monoclonal antibodies to the p21 products of the
transforming gene of Harvey murine sarcoma virus and of
the cellular ras gene family. J. Virology: 43: 294-330.
Heilig, R., Perrin, F., Gannon, F., Mandel, J.L., Chambon,
P., 1980. The ovalbumin gene family: structure of the
X gene and evolution of duplicated split genes. Cell 20:
625-637.
Parada, L.F., Jabin, C.J., Shih, C., and Weinberg, R.A.,
1982. Human EJ bladder carcinoma oncogene is homologue
of Harvey sarcoma virus ras gene. Nature 297: 474-478.

Scolnick, E.M., Weeks, M.O., Shih, T.Y., Ruscetti, S.K. and Dexter, T.M., 1981. Markedly elevated levels of an endo-genous sarc protein in a hemopoietic precursor cell line. Molecular and Cellular Biology 1: 66-74.

Setzer, D.R., McGrogan, M., Nunberg, J.H., and Schimke, R.T., 1980. Size heterogeneity in the 3' end of dihydrofolate reductase messenger RNAs in mouse cells. Cell 22: 361-370.

Shih, T.Y., Weeks, M.O., Young, H.A., and Scolnick, E.M., 1979. Identification of a sarcoma virus coded phosphopro-tein in nonproducer cells transformed by Kirsten or Harvey murine sarcoma virus. Virology 96: 64-79.

Shih, T.Y., Weeks, M.O., Gruss, P., Dhar, R., Oroszlan, S., and Scolnick, E.M., 1982. Identification of a precursor in the biosynthesis of the p21 transforming protein of Harvey murine sarcoma virus. J. Virology 42: 253-261.

Tsuchida, N., Ryder, T., and Ohtsubo, E., 1982. Nucleotide sequence of Kirsten murine sarcoma virus oncogene coding for p21 transforming protein. Science: 217: 948-951.

Oncogenes and Retroviruses: Evaluation of Basic Findings
and Clinical Potential, pages 79–90
© 1983 Alan R. Liss, Inc., 150 Fifth Avenue, New York, NY 10011

TUMORIGENESIS BY TRANSFECTED CELLS IN NUDE MICE: A NEW
METHOD FOR DETECTING CELLULAR TRANSFORMING GENES

D. G. Blair[1], C. S. Cooper[2], M. K. Oskarsson[2],
L. A. Eader[3], and G. F. Vande Woude[2]

[1]Laboratory of Molecular Oncology, National
Cancer Institute, Frederick, MD 21701,
[2]Laboratory of Molecular Oncology, National
Cancer Institute, Bethesda, MD 20205, and
[3]NIH Intramural Research Support Program,
NCI-Frederick Cancer Research Facility,
Frederick, MD 21701

The neoplastic transformation of normal cells induces
complex changes at the phenotypic, biochemical and molecular levels. While these changes involve large numbers of
specific cellular functions, it has been known for some
time that initiation and maintenance of these alterations
can be due to the presence and expression in transformed
cells of relatively small amounts of specific, genetic
information. DNA viruses such as polyoma and SV40 and
RNA viruses such as Rous sarcoma virus and Moloney sarcoma
virus, contain genes whose insertion into cellular DNA,
and subsequent expression, leads to cell transformation.
Oncogenic viral models have led to the hypothesis that
other non-viral transformation events might be due to
the expression of dominant endogenous transforming genes
whose transforming potential is triggered by some
primary oncogenic event. However, direct evidence for
such dominant cellular transforming genes as the cause
of non-viral transformation has been lacking.

Recently though, advances in techniques of gene
transfer has led to the identification and isolation of
specific gene sequences present in spontaneous and
chemically-transformed cells of both animal and human
origin (Shih et al., 1979; Cooper et al., 1980; Krontiris

and Cooper, 1981; Shih et al., 1981; Lane et al., 1981;
Murry et al., 1981; Perucho et al., 1981; Hopkins et al.,
1981; Lane et al., 1982; Shih and Weinberg, 1982; Pulcioni
et al., 1982, Goldfarb et al., 1982) which are capable
of exerting dominant transforming effects when introduced
into normal, non-transformed cells. The identification
of such sequences has been based, with few exceptions
(Hopkins et al., 1981; Smith et al., 1982), on their
ability to induce morphologically-transformed foci on
NIH 3T3 cells, a flat fibroblastic line derived from NIH
Swiss mice (Todaro and Green, 1963). The ability of
these cells to register such transformation events
efficiently is variable, sensitive to a variety of cell
culture conditions, and often requires subjective judg-
ments to initially differentiate transformed foci from
spontaneous morphological changes in the cell monolayer.
In addition, the microscopic screening of large numbers
of tissue culture dishes represents a time-consuming and
tedious task. These considerations, coupled with our
belief that some neoplastic transformation events might
not involve a readily distinguishable change in cell
morphology, led us to consider alternative methods of
selection and enrichment for transformed cells in a
transfected cell population.

The ability of cells to form progressively growing
tumors when injected into athymic nu/nu (nude) mice is
a relatively definitive demonstration of the neoplastic
state (Fogh and Giovanella, 1978). Furthermore, the
selective pressures exerted on a cell population during
the formation of a tumor might result in the selection
of a set of transforming genes in a tumor different from
those selected during the formation of a morphologically-
transformed focus. For these reasons we chose to evaluate
the potential of the nude mouse as a vehicle for detecting and selecting transformed cells from a population of
cells transfected with dominant oncogenes. The results
we present here indicate that such a procedure can be
used to detect dominant cellular transforming genes,
including those present in transformed human cell lines,
and that this method represents a useful alternative to
the standard focus induction assay as a means of identifying and isolating such genes.

Tumor Induction by Cells Transfected by Viral
Oncogenes: We initially measured the ability of cells
transfected with various amounts of the molecularly
cloned provirus of Moloney sarcoma virus (MSV), an acute
transforming retrovirus (Vande Woude et al., 1979) to
induce tumors in nude mice.

Table 1 shows that mice injected with MSV-transfected
cells developed tumors 6–8 weeks after injection. Aliquots of transfected cells were also maintained in tissue
culture and foci were counted 14 days later. In these
experiments, the MSV DNA had a specific activity of 9000
focus forming units per µg of cloned DNA. The results
suggest that cells transfected with even small amounts
of MSV DNA could induce tumors in nude mice. At higher
DNA levels more tumors were induced and the tumors arose
more quickly. The fact that only 4 of 5 mice developed
tumors at the highest DNA level tested was unexpected,
but it could reflect the T-cell independent anti-tumor
cell response known to be present in nude mice (Herberman
et al., 1975). These and other experiments suggested,
however, that tumor induction by MSV-transfected cells
was as sensitive as focus formation in detecting transformed cells in a transfected cell population. The
tumors arose at the site of injection and appeared to be
undifferentiated fibrosarcomas (K. Stromberg, personal
communication). Infectious MSV could be rescued by
Moloney murine leukemia virus superinfection of tumor
cell derived cell lines (4 rescuable of 8 tested). This
proportion of MSV rescue is similar to that observed for
lines derived from foci induced by MSV in conventional
DNA transfections (Blair et al., 1980).

As a further measure of the sensitivity of the
assay, we examined whether cell DNA isolated from virally-
transformed cell lines could be detected in the assay.
High molecular weight cellular DNA was isolated from an
MSV-transformed mink lung cell line (HTMF, Vande Woude
et al., 1979) and from an SV40-transformed human cell
line (SV80, Todaro and Meyer, 1974). NIH 3T3 cells were
transfected with 100 µg of each of these DNA preparations,
and 24 hrs later the cells were divided into 5 aliquots
and injected into nude mice. In 3 separate experiments
with HTMF DNA, a total of 5 of 14 mice injected developed

Table 1. Tumor Formation by NIH 3T3 Cells Transfected with Cloned λml MSV DNA

	Injected per Mouse		Fraction Tumors Induced	Tumor Appearance (Wks. after Inj.)
	DNA Equiv.[a]	Cells[b]		
Exp. 1	400	8×10^5	4/5	6
	40	7×10^5	4/5	7
	4	3×10^5	2/3	7
	0.4	4×10^5	1/5	8
	---	3×10^5	0/4	18
Exp. 2	4	1×10^6	2/4	9
	0.4	1×10^6	0/10	16
		1×10^6	0/10	16
	---	1×10^6	0/5	16

[a] 5×10^6 NIH 3T3 cells were transfected as previously described (Blair et al., 1980) with EcoR1 restricted λml MSV DNA, containing the indicated amount of proviral DNA, in the presence of 20 μg of calf thymus DNA as carrier. Cells were trypsinized, washed and injected into mice approximately 18 hours later.

[b] The indicated number of cells was injected in 0.1 ml of serum-free Dulbecco's modified minimum essential medium.

[c] Number of mice developing tumors/total number of mice injected.

tumors, while in one experiment with SV80 DNA, 3 of 5 mice developed tumors. In both cases the tumors were first detected from 5-7 weeks after injection. MSV could be rescued from 2 of 3 cell lines derived from HTMF DNA-induced tumors, while SV40 T antigen was detected by immunofluorescence utilizing anti-SV40 T antisera in the 3 cell lines derived from the SV80 DNA-induced tumors. These results strongly suggested that the tumors arose as the result of the transfer of SV40 and MSV genetic sequences, and indicated that the assay was sensitive enough to detect transforming genes present at low copy number in the genomes of transformed cells.

Tumor Induction by Cells Transfected with Transformed Human Cell DNA: To determine if tumor induction by nude mice could be used to detect transforming sequences present in transformed human cell lines, DNA was prepared from several human cell lines, transfected into NIH 3T3 cells, and these cells were injected into nude mice. As indicated in Table 2, cells transfected by 3 of 6 DNAs tested were able to induce tumors in nude mice in 5-8 weeks. This suggested that the human pancreatic carconoma-derived cell line (A1165) (Lieber et al., 1975) the human fibrosarcoma-derived cell line (HT 1080) (Rasheed et al., 1974) and the chemically-transformed human osteosarcoma derived cell line (MNNG-HOS) (Rhim et al., 1975) contained dominant transforming genes. For purposes of comparison to the nude mouse assay, the ability of each of the DNA samples to induce foci in the conventional focus induction DNA transfection assay was also tested. The pancreatic carcinoma DNA transformed with efficiencies of 0.35-0.67 focus forming units per μg (ffu/μg), while the MNNG-HOS DNA had an efficiency of 0.02-0.10 ffu/μg. We were unable to detect any foci on cells transfected with 100 μg of HT 1080 fibrosarcoma DNA, although others have reported a low level of activity for DNA prepared from this cell line (Pulciani et al., 1982). Since tumors were induced when cells transfected in these same experiments were injected into mice, this suggests that in some cases the tumor induction assay may detect transformation events not detectable in the conventional focus assay.

As has been demonstrated by several investigators (Murry et al., 1981; Perucho et al., 1981; Lane et al., 1982; Shih and Weinberg, 1982; Pulciani et al., 1982), transformed cells induced by transfection of human cell DNA contain human genetic sequences. These sequences are readily detectable in Southern blots (Southern, 1975) of restriction endonuclease digested DNA by hybridization to probes containing human highly repeated sequences. Accordingly we examined EcoRl digested DNAs from tumors and foci induced by human cell DNA transfection for the presence of DNA sequences homologous to probe prepared from Blur 8 (Jelinck et al., 1980), a clone containing a member of the alu family of highly repeated human DNA. Normal NIH 3T3 DNA did not hybridize to the probe, but the primary tumor induced by A1165 DNA, as well as tumors

induced by MNNG–HOS DNA and HT 1080 DNA showed extensive
hybridization. Three tumors which arose after injection
of HT 1080 DNA did not contain alu hybridizable sequences,
suggesting that these tumors may have arisen spontaneously
and not as a direct result of human DNA uptake. Alu positive tumor DNA contains large numbers of hybridizing bands,
and no definite conclusions can be drawn as to the presence of common bands in either tumors or foci. It does
appear, however, that independent tumors and foci show
different banding patterns, while DNA isolated from a
tumor explant shows a banding pattern similar to the DNA
of the tumor from which it was isolated.

As indicated in Table 2, cells transfected with
DNA of several other human transformed cell lines also
induced tumors. These tumors arose late (at 9–15 weeks
after injection) and those we have examined do not
contain detectable levels of human alu sequences.
These include a human melanoma line (A1589), a human
bladder carcinoma line (A1663), a human teratocarcinoma
line (Hu Ter 1; Fogh and Toempe, 1975) and a chemically-
transformed human fibroblast line (HUT 14; Kakunaga,
1978).

To test the hypothesis that the acquired human
sequences were reponsible for the tumor induction, DNA
prepared from the mouse tumor was used to induce secondary
foci and tumors. Data obtained from analysis of 4 primary
and 1 secondary tumor is shown in Table 3. Both human
pancreatic carcinoma induced tumor DNAs (A1165) induced
both foci and mouse tumors in several independent experiments. Analysis of DNA from several of these secondary
tumors showed the presence of alu hybridizing sequences
and several secondary foci also showed alu hybridizing
bands (data not shown). The pattern observed in the
foci suggested that they may contain alu hybridizing
fragments of similar size. The patterns observed in
secondary tumors were complex, however, and no clear conclusions could be drawn. DNA obtained from two primary
MNNG–HOS-induced tumors also induced foci in secondary
transfections, although the second tumor exhibited only
a low focus forming activity and no tumors were induced.

Table 2. Transforming Activity of Human Tumor-Derived Cell Line DNA

Cell Line Designation	Origin	Focus Formation (per µg)	Tumors (No. Tumors / No. Mice inj.)	Tumor Appearance (Wks)	Human Repeat Sequences[a]
Al165	Human pancreatic carconima	0.35-0.67	1/5	6	1/1
CCL 121	Human fibrosarcoma (HT 1080)	<0.01[b]	5/5	5-9	2/5
CRL-1574	Chemically-transformed human osteosarcoma (MNNG-HOS)	0.05	3/5	5	3/3
HUT 14	Chemically-transformed human fibroblast	NT[c]	0/10	-	-
Al589	Human melanoma	<0.01	1/5	15	0/1
Al663	Human bladder carcinoma	NT	2/5	10,15	0/1
Hu Tera1	Human tetracarcinoma	<0.01	3/5	9,11	0/1

a Detected by hybridization of human alu repeat family Blur 8 clone probe to Southern blots of EcoRl-digested tumor DNA.
b No foci detected in cells transfected with 100 µg.
c Not tested.

Table 3.   Tumors and foci induced by secondary and
           tertiary mouse tumor DNA from human DNA
           transfections

Primary Tumor[a] Induced by	Foci Induced per μg DNA	Tumors Induced	Tumor Appearance (Wks)
A1165–T1	0.1–5.0	9/10	4–7
A1165–T1 animal transplant	0.1–0.6	3/15	5,7
MNNG–HOS–T1	0.05	6/10	4–7,10
MNNG–HOS–T2	0.01	0/5	10
A1165 secondary tumor MT-84	0.3–0.6	–––	–––

[a]DNA isolated from the tumors indicated was analyzed in
both focus and tumor induction assays as described
above. Each mouse was injected with cells transfected
by 20μg of cell DNA.

Tumor Induction by Normal NIH 3T3 Cells: We have
measured the ability of morphologically normal NIH 3T3
cells, as well as NIH 3T3 cells transfected with a variety
of high molecular weight DNAs derived from non-neoplastic
cells and tissues (calf thymus, human placenta, E. coli,
NIH 3T3 mouse cells), to form tumors when injected subcutaneously into BALB/c nude mice. In most cases, injection
of between 10^6 and 10^7 cells does not result in tumor
formation, although we have observed a low incidence of
tumors arising 10 or more weeks after injection with
both transfected and non-transfected cells (two tumors
in 76 mice). In a few cases, however, we have observed
a high incidence of early (3-6 weeks) tumor induction in
cells transfected with non-neoplastic DNA, but these
appear to be due to spontaneous changes in particular
cell cultures, and occur only infrequently. The use of
low passage cells 1-2 passages after revival from nitrogen
storage, coupled with the injection of 1-2 x 10^6 cells
per mouse has minimized the occurrence of such "background"
tumors. In addition, since our data indicates that tumors

induced by cells transfected with transforming DNA appears
to arise within 4-8 weeks of cell injection, we generally
view tumors arising 10 or more weeks after injection as
likely to be due to non-transfection related events.

Summary and Conclusion:

We have demonstrated that NIH 3T3 cells freshly
transfected with either a cloned retroviral provirus or
cell DNA derived from virally-transformed cells are able
to induce tumors when injected subcutaneously into nude
mice. Furthermore, cells transfected with DNA derived
from at least three transformed human cell lines are
able to induce tumors. These latter tumors contain
human DNA sequences and DNA isolated from at least some
of them is able to induce both foci and tumors in subsequent DNA transfection. Our data suggests that tumor
induction by transfected 3T3 cells could serve as a
powerful system for the selection of cells transformed
by dominant cellular oncogenes. This method oviates the
requirement that oncogenes induce clearly defined
morphologically-transformed foci in order to be detected,
and eliminates the need to maintain morphologically
normal cells in tissue culture for many weeks, as well
as the necessity of microscopically screning large numbers
of tissue culture dishes. The tumors which arise in
nude mice grow progressively, have been readily trans-
plantable to other nude mice, and have been readily
explantable into tissue culture. In addition, both DNA
and RNA can be isolated directly from the mouse tumors
to screen for the presence and expression of transfected
sequences.

We are currently examining other DNA samples from
both human tumor-derived cell lines and primary human
tumors to determine if this assay will detect and identify additional oncogenes. We are also studying the
suitability of other normal cell lines as recipients in
this assay, since cell lines which do not show readily
discernible morphological transformation in monolayer
culture may be suitable as tumor inducers following
transfection. This assay should provide a convenient
alternative method for detecting transforming genes and
may help to increase the number of such sequence which
can be identified and analyzed.

Acknowledgments:

   We wish to thank J. DeLarco, J. S. Rhim, T. Kakemaga
and P. J. Fischinger for providing transformed human
cell lines used in these studies, and K. Stromberg for
the histological analysis of various tumor samples. We
also wish to thank S. Showalter and K. Dunn for their
expert technical assistance, and K. Cannon for preparing
the manuscript for publication.

References:

Blair DG, McClements WL, Oskarsson M, Fischinger PJ, and
   Vande Woude GF (1980). Biological activity of cloned
   Moloney sarcoma virus DNA: Terminally redundant sequences
   may enhance transformation efficiency. Proc Natl Acad
   Sci USA 77:3504.
Cooper GM, Okenquist S, and Silverman LA (1980). Trans-
   forming activity of DNA of chemically-transformed and
   normal cells. Nature 284:418.
Fogh J and Tempe, G (1975).
   In Fogh J (ed): "Human Tumors In Vitro", New York:
   Plenum Press, p 115.
Giovanella BC and Fogh J (1978). Present and future
   trends in investigations with the nude mouse as a
   recipient of human tumor transplants. In Fogh J and
   Giovanella BC (eds): "The Nude Mouse in Experimental
   and Clinical Research", Vol 1, New York, Academic
   Press, p 281.
Goldfarb M, Shimiza K, Perucho M, and Wigler M (1982).
   Isolation and preliminary characterization of a human
   transforming gene from T24 bladder carcinoma cells.
   Nature 296:404.
Herberman RB, Numa ME, and Lansing DH (1975). Natural
   cytotoxic reactivity of mouse lymphoid cells against
   syngeneic and allogeneic tumors. I. Distribution of
   reactivity and specificity. Int J Cancer 16:216.
Hopkins N, Besmer P, DeLeo AB, and Law, LW (1981).
   High frequency cotransfer of the transformed phenotype and a tumor-specific transplantation antigen
   by DNA from the 3-methylcholantrine-induced Meth A
   sarcoma of BALB/c mice. Proc Natl Acad Sci USA 78:
   7555.

Jelnick WR, Toomey TP, Leinwod L, Duncan CH, Biro, PA, Choudary PV, Weissman SM, Rabin CM, Houck CM, Deininger PL, and Schmid CW (1980). Ubiquitous, interspersed repeated sequences in mammalian genomes. Proc Natl Acad Sci USA 77:1398.

Kakunaga T (1978). Neoplastic transformation of human diploid fibroblast cells by chemical carcinogens. Proc Natl Acad Sci USA 75:1334.

Krontiris TG and Cooper GM (1981). Transforming activity of human tumor DNAs. Proc Natl Acad Sci USA 78:1181.

Lane MA, Sainten A, and Cooper GM (1981). Activation of related transforming genes in mouse and human mammary carcinogens. Proc Natl Acad Sci USA 78:5185.

Lane MA, Sainten A, and Cooper GM (1982). Stage-specific transforming genes of human and mouse B- and T-lymphocyte neoplasms. Cell 28:873.

Lieber M, Mayzetta J, Nelson-Rees W, Kaplan M, and Todaro G (1975). Establishment of a continuous tumor-cell line (Panc-1) from a human carcinoma of the exocrine pancreas. Int J Cancer 15:741.

Murry M, Shilo B, Shih C, Cowing D, Hsu HW, and Weinberg RA (1981). Three different human tumor lines contain different oncogenes. Cell 25:355.

Perucho M, Goldfarb M, Shimizu K, Lama C, Fogh J, and Wigler M (1981). Human tumor-derived cell lines contain common and different transforming genes. Cell 27:467.

Pulciani S, Santos E, Lauver AV, Long LK, Robbins KC, and Barbacid M (1982). Oncogenes in human tumor cell lines: Molecular cloning of a transforming gene from human bladder carcinoma cells. Proc Natl Acad Sci USA 79:2845.

Rasheed S, Nelson-Rees WA, Toth EM, Arnstein P, and Gardner MB (1974). Characterization of a newly-derived human sarcoma cell line (HT 1080). Cancer 33:1027.

Rhim JS, Park DK, Arnstein P, Huebner RJ, Weisburger EK, and Nelson-Rees WA (1975). Transformation of human cells in culture by N-methyl-N'-nitro-N-nitrosoguanidine. Nature 256:751.

Shih C, Padhy LC, Murray M, and Weinberg RA (1981). Transforming genes of carcinomas and neuroblastomas introduced into mouse fibroblasts. Nature 290:261.

Shih C, Shilo BZ, Goldfarb MP, Dannenberg A, and
  Weinberg RA (1979). Passage of phenotypes of
  chemically-transformed cells via transfection of
  DNA and chromatin. Proc Natl Acad Sci USA 76:5714.
Shih C and Weinberg RA (1982). Isolation of a trans-
  forming sequence from a human bladder carcinoma cell
  line. Cell 29:161.
Smith BL, Anesowicz A, Chodosh LA, and Sager R (1982).
  DNA transfer of focus- and tumor-forming ability
  into non-tumorigenic CHEF cells. Proc Natl Acad
  Sci USA 79:1964.
Southern EM (1975). Detection of specific sequences
  among DNA fragments separated by gel electrophoresis.
  J Mol Biol 98:503.
Todaro GJ and Meyer CA (1974). Transformation assay
  for murine sarcoma viruses using a Simian virus 40
  transformed human cell line. J Natl Cancer Inst 52:
  167.
Todaro GJ and Green H (1963). Quantitative studies on
  the growth of mouse embryo cells in culture and their
  development into established lines. J Cell Biol 17:
  299.
Vande Woude GF, Oskarsson M, Enquist LW, Nomura A,
  Sullivan M, and Fischinger PJ (1979). Cloning of
  integrated Moloney sarcoma proviral DNA sequences
  in bacteriophage λ. Proc Natl Acad Sci USA 76:4464.

ONCOGENE: CHROMOSOMAL LOCALIZATION AND FUNCTION

Oncogenes and Retroviruses: Evaluation of Basic Findings
and Clinical Potential, pages 93–103
© 1983 Alan R. Liss, Inc., 150 Fifth Avenue, New York, NY 10011

GENETIC ORGANIZATION OF HUMAN PROTO-ONCOGENES

Alan Y. Sakaguchi, Ph.D.

Department of Human Genetics
Roswell Park Memorial Institute
Buffalo, N.Y. 14263

More than a dozen normal cellular genes have served as
progenitors for oncogenes of acute transforming retroviruses
of mammals and birds (see review by Bishop 1982). The
presence of proto-oncogenes in uninfected cells and their
evolutionary conservation in widely divergent phylogenetic
species have suggested important roles in normal cellular
and organismal biochemistry (Barnekow et al. 1982; Roussel
et al. 1979; Shilo, Weinberg 1981; Spector et al. 1978;
Stehelin et al. 1976). Recent findings from a number of
laboratories have implicated several proto-oncogenes in
malignant transformation of cells (see review by Cooper
1982), indicating that under certain circumstances normal
cellular genes may acquire oncogenic potency. Those
observations provide a motive and rationale for determining
if proto-oncogenes are located on chromosomes whose
numerical or structural aberrations are frequently associated
with certain forms of cancer (see review by Rowley, Testa
1982). This article reviews our efforts begun approximately
two years ago aimed at determining the genetic organization
of proto-oncogenes principally in man, but also in mouse.
These studies have relied largely upon interspecies somatic
cell hybrids (Weiss, Green 1967) and Southern blot
hybridization techniques (Southern 1975).

DETECTING CELLULAR PROTO-ONCOGNES

Molecular clones of retrovirus oncogenes have been
useful for detecting homologous sequences in host cell
genomic DNA and cytoplasmic RNA (Bishop 1982). Used in

conjunction with blot hybridization techniques, these probes allow the detection of homologous genes occurring once per haploid cellular genome. It has been possible to chromosomally assign proto-oncogenes in man and mouse with an *in vitro* parasexual genetic approach employing interspecies somatic cell hybrids. DNA from man-mouse hybrids (losing human chromosomes) and mouse-Chinese hamster hybrids (losing mouse chromosomes) can be analyzed for the presence of proto-oncogenes using cloned viral or cellular oncogene probes. The particular human or mouse chromosomes present in hybrids can be determined by assaying for previously assigned genetic markers and by direct karyotyping (Shows et al. 1982). The segregation of unique proto-oncogene bands on blots can be shown to coincide with a particular chromosome in cell hybrids.

CHROMOSOME ASSIGNMENT OF PROTO-ONCOGENES

Table 1 lists some of the human and mouse proto-oncogenes we have assigned to date. Two of the human proto-oncogenes, c-*src* and c-*myc*, were detected using cloned probes of v-*src* and v-*myc*, the oncogenes of Rous sarcoma virus, and avian myelocytomatosis virus MC29, respectively (provided by JM Bishop and colleagues).

Table 1. Chromosome Assignment of Human and Mouse
Proto-oncogenes

Proto-oncogene	Probe	Enzyme	Size fragments(kb) Human/Mouse	Chromosome Human/Mouse	
c-*src*	pSRA-2 (JM Bishop)	EcoRI	28/14,15.5	20	2
c-Ki-*ras*-2	p640 (RA Weinberg)	EcoRI	2.9	12	?
c-*myc*	pVMYC-3-Pst (JM Bishop)	HindIII	10.8/4.4	8	15

Proto-oncogenes were assigned using the molecular clones listed. DNAs from somatic cell hybrids were cleaved with the indicated restriction enzyme and analyzed by blot hybridization (Sakaguchi et al. 1982). Sizes of specific hybridizing fragments of human and mouse DNA are given.

The third proto-oncogene listed in Table 1 had a different origin. Colon c-onc (a generic name only) was

isolated from SW480 human colonic adenocarcinoma cells using
a combination of DNA-mediated transfection and molecular
cloning techniques (see review by Weinberg 1982). DNA
transfection experiments of Weinberg and colleagues
indicated that SW480 harbored a gene capable of inducing
oncogenic transformation of mouse NIH 3T3 cells. This human
gene, isolated by molecular cloning methods, has been
identified as a cellular homolog (c-Ki-*ras*-2) of the
oncogene of Kirsten murine sarcoma virus, v-Ki-*ras*
(RA Weinberg personal communication). An identical transforming gene has also been detected in at least five other
independently derived human colon and lung carcinoma cells.
Moreover, the activated cellular transforming gene of the
human EJ bladder carcinoma cell line is now known to be a
cellular homolog of the oncogene of Harvey sarcoma virus,
v-Ha-*ras*-1 (Der et al. 1982; Parada et al. 1982).

Each proto-oncogene was chromosomally assigned by
analyzing the DNA from more than 30 human-mouse cell hybrids.
In each instance a specific hybridizing DNA fragment
heralded the presence of the proto-oncogene in a given
hybrid clone. Hybrid cells were also karyotyped to confirm
the assignment by enzyme marker analysis. The assignments
of c-*src*, c-*myc*, and colon c-onc are summarized in Table 1,
and each will be described individually below.

A human c-*src* gene was detected by its ability to
hybridize with the v-*src* gene of Rous sarcoma virus, an
avian retrovirus. Bishop and colleagues had previously
demonstrated the presence of *src* sequences in all vertebrates
examined, including human and mouse, using liquid hybridization techniques (Spector et al. 1978; Stehelin et al. 1976).
We were able to detect human and mouse c-*src* genes by
Southern hybridization, and could demonstrate unique
hybridizing DNA fragments using the restriction endonuclease
EcoRI (Sakaguchi et al. 1982). In human DNA the v-*src* probe
hybridized principally to a 28 kbp EcoRI DNA fragment, which
was easily distinguished from the 14 and 15.5 kbp fragments
of mouse DNA hybridizing with v-*src*. The human c-*src* gene
was assigned to chromosome 20 by its concordant segregation
with the chromosome 20 marker adenosine deaminase, and with
a karyotypically normal chromosome 20 (Sakaguchi et al. 1982).

A second human proto-oncogene was detected using a
probe containing v-*myc*, the oncogene of avian myelocytomatosis virus MC29 (probe pVMYC-3-Pst from JM Bishop and

colleagues). MC29 is another example of an acute transforming retrovirus possessing a cell-derived oncogene (Roussel
et al. 1979; Sheiness, Bishop 1979). Human and mouse DNAs
cleaved with HindIII yield DNA fragments of approximately
10.8 and 4.4 kbp, respectively, that hybridize to v-*myc*.
The 10.8 kbp human c-*myc* sequence segregated in hybrids
concordantly with the human chromosome 8 marker glutathione
reductase, and with a karyotypically normal chromosome 8
(Sakaguchi et al. manuscript in preparation).

Using the p640 colon c-onc probe, the c-Ki-*ras*-2 gene
was assigned to human chromosome 12 (Sakaguchi et al.
manuscript in preparation). p640 detected a single 2.9 kbp
EcoRI fragment of human DNA which segregated in cell hybrids
concordantly with the human chromosome 12 enzyme markers
lactate dehydrogenase-B and peptidase-B. The Kirsten and
Harvey v-*ras* genes are thought to be derived from divergent
members of a multigene family (Ellis et al. 1981). It is
of interest to note, therefore, that the c-Ha-*ras*-1 proto-
oncogene which is related to c-Ki-*ras*-2 has been assigned
to human chromosome 11 (de Martinville et al. submitted for
publication).

The three proto-oncogenes discussed here share some
common characteristics. All appear to occupy constant
chromosome locations (cell hybrids were derived from a dozen
unrelated human parental cells). Since all human-mouse
hybrids used were derived from cells from normal individuals,
the chromosome assignments represent the native proto-
oncogene locations. A survey of more than 20 DNAs from
normal human fibroblasts and leukocytes has not revealed
any marked difference in gene copy number for any of the
three proto-oncogenes. However, amplification of proto-
oncogenes has been observed in some human and animal tumor
cells (Collins, Groudine 1982; Dalla-Favera et al. 1982a;
Noori-Daloii et al. 1981) and also in certain strains of
mouse (Chattopadhyay et al. 1982).

CHROMOSOME ASSIGNMENT OF MOUSE PROTO-ONCOGENES

Our interests also include the genetic organization of
proto-oncogenes in the mouse. Accordingly, a collection of
15 Chinese hamster-mouse cell hybrids losing mouse chromosomes were utilized to chromosomally assign mouse proto-
oncogenes (in collaboration with PA Lalley). DNAs from

cell hybrid lines were analyzed by blot hybridization using the restriction enzymes and cloned oncogene probes listed in Table 1. Mouse c-*src* and c-*myc* sequences were assigned to chromosomes 2 and 15, respectively (Sakaguchi et al. manuscript in preparation).

These chromosome assignments are of interest not only with regard to the evolutionary history of proto-oncogenes, but also in relationship to chromosome abnormalities in tumor cells (discussed later).

POSSIBLE CONSERVATION OF PROTO-ONCOGENE LINKAGE GROUPS

Certain genes in man and mouse have remained linked during the 80 million years of evolution separating these two species (see Lalley et al. 1978 and Shows et al. 1982 for a discussion of this topic and references). For example, five genes in the mouse (*Eno*-1, *Pgd*, *Pgm*-2, *Ak*-2, and *Gpd*-1) are located on chromosome 4. All the human homologs of these five genes are located on the short arm of human chromosome 1. A comparison of the locations of mouse and human c-*src* suggest that this proto-oncogene might also reside in a conserved linkage group (Table 2). Along with human c-*src* (Sakaguchi et al. 1982), the genes coding for inosine triphosphatase and adenosine deaminase have been assigned to chromosome 20 (Hopkinson et al. 1975; Meera Khan et al. 1975; Tischfield et al. 1974). Mouse inosine triphosphatase is located on chromosome 2, also the probable site for mouse adenosine deaminase (PA Lalley unpublished data). Inosine triphosphatase was assigned using Chinese hamster-mouse cell hybrids, whereas adenosine deaminase was assigned using mouse-human hybrids segregating mouse chromosomes. Thus, these three genes in man and mouse might represent a conserved linkage group. Regional localization of these markers in both species should further clarify their evolutionary relationships.

Table 2. Comparative Assignment of c-*src* in Man and Mouse

Marker	Chromosome Location	
	Human	Mouse
c-*src*	20	2
Adenosine deaminase	20	2
Inosine triphosphatase	20	2

Presently, there are insufficient markers on human chromosome 8 to decide whether mouse and human c-*myc* might reside in a conserved linkage group. However, the assignment of c-*myc* genes to human chromosome 8 and mouse chromosome 15 may bear an important relationship to structural abnormalities involving these chromosomes in lymphoid neoplasms (Klein 1981; Rowley, Testa 1982).

PROTO-ONCOGENES, CHROMOSOME TRANSLOCATIONS, AND NEOPLASIA

The assignment of human and mouse c-*myc* genes to chromosomes 8 and 15, respectively, is of interest as numerical and structural abnormalities of these chromosomes occur frequently in certain hematopoietic malignancies in the two species (Klein 1981; Rowley, Testa 1982). For example, a translocation of a portion of chromosome 8 (q24) to chromosomes 2, 14, or 22 in some Burkitt's lymphomas and B-cell derived acute lymphocytic leukemias have been described (Rowley, Testa 1982). The human genes for immunoglobulin heavy chains are located on chromosome 14 (Croce et al. 1979) and have been localized to the region of 14 involved in the 8;14 translocation seen in some BL cell lines (Kirsch et al. 1982).

In a recent survey of 19 Burkitt's lymphoma cell lines, each carrying one of three translocations involving chromosome 8 (8;14, 2;8, or 8;22), Lenoir et al. (1982) have reported that λ and κ light chain production was specific for cells carrying the 8;22 and 2;8 translocations, respectively. These results suggest (but do not prove) that the immunoglobulin gene loci on the translocations have become activated. An apparently analogous situation occurs in mouse plasmacytomas in which specific 6;15 and 12;15 translocations are associated with κ and λ light chain expression, respectively (Klein 1981). The mouse κ and heavy immunoglobulin genes occur on chromosomes 6 and 12, respectively (D'Eustachio et al. 1980; Swan et al. 1979). The occurrence of specific translocations involving chromosomes bearing immunoglobulin genes has fostered speculation that genes involved in B cell proliferation have become activated because of their juxtaposition to immunoglobulin gene regions that undergo rearrangement during B cell differentiation (Klein 1981). The possibility that these non-immunoglobulin gene regions may harbor proto-oncogenes has also been suggested (Klein 1981; Pall 1981). To resolve these questions, we are currently localizing human and mouse c-*myc* genes using several approaches, including translocation chromosomes and high resolution *in situ* hybridization techniques (Zabel et al. 1982).

Elevated expression of c-*myc* in at least two species (chickens and humans) has been observed (Dalla-Favera et al. 1982a; Hayward et al. 1981; Payne et al. 1982) and appears to involve different mechanisms. In approximately 80% of B-lymphomas of chickens induced by lymphoid leukosis virus, viral DNA sequences are inserted near the c-*myc* gene (Hayward et al. 1981). Enhanced transcription of c-*myc* is believed to be initiated from the viral promoter in the lymphoma cells. This phenomenon has been termed "oncogenesis by promoter insertion" (Hayward et al. 1981). Avian syncytia virus also appears to integrate near c-*myc* in chicken B-cell lymphomas (Fung et al. 1981).

The HL60 line of malignant promyelocytes from a patient with acute promyelocytic leukemia contains multiple c-*myc* genes, amplified in copy number roughly 16-fold (Collins, Groudine 1982; Dalla-Favera et al. 1982a). HL60 cells also contain an elevated level of c-*myc* RNA transcripts that is consistent with the observed gene amplification (Dalla-Favera et al. 1982a). Amplification of c-*myc* genes in chicken B-cell lymphomas has also been observed (Noori-Daloii et al. 1981).

The exact role that elevated expression of c-*myc* might play in the malignant phenotype of cancer cells is not presently clear. However, it should be of interest to determine if elevated c-*myc* expression in certain Burkitt's lymphoma cell lines (AY Sakaguchi unpublished data) can be related at the molecular level with the presence of the 8;14 translocation.

EPILOGUE

The proto-oncogenes discussed here and those studied by other groups (Dalla-Favera et al. 1982b; Swan et al. 1982) reflect the rapid progress being made at constructing a chromosome map of human and mouse proto-oncogenes. These initial reports engender optimism that soon the chromosomal locations of all presently known proto-oncogenes will be determined. We believe that chromosome assignment of proto-oncogenes will yield useful information concerning not only their relationships to chromosome abnormalities associated with certain forms of cancer, but also their evolutionary histories.

ACKNOWLEDGMENTS

I wish to acknowledge the contributions of my collaborators TB Shows, PA Lalley, SL Naylor, and RA Weinberg and colleagues. I wish to thank JM Bishop and colleagues for the cloned retrovirus oncogenes, and CR Young for preparing the manuscript.

This work was supported in part by funds from the American Cancer Society (Institutional Grant IN54T-21), Biomedical Research Support Grants, and a USPHS grant GM 20454.

REFERENCES

Barnekow A, Schartl M, Anders F, Bauer H (1982). Identifi- cation of a fish protein associated with a kinase activity and related to the Rous sarcoma virus transforming protein. Cancer Res 42:2429.
Bishop JM (1982). Oncogenes. Scientific American 246:80.
Chattopadhyay SK, Chang EH, Lander MR, Ellis RW, Scolnick EM, Lowy DR (1982). Amplification and rearrange- ment of onc genes in mammalian species. Nature 296:361.
Collins S, Groudine M. (1982). Amplification of endogenous myc-related DNA sequences in a human myeloid leukemia cell line. Nature 298:679.
Cooper GM (1982). Cellular transforming genes. Science 218:801.
Croce CM, Shander M, Martinis J, Cicurel L, D'Ancona GG, Colby TW, Koprowski H (1979). Chromosomal location of the genes for human immunoglobulin heavy chains. Proc Natl Acad Sci USA 76:2735.
Dalla Favera R, Wong-Staal F, Gallo RC (1982a). onc gene amplification in promyelocytic leukaemia cell line HL-60 and primary leukaemic cells of the same patient. Nature 299:61.
Dalla-Favera R, Franchini G, Martinotti S, Wong-Staal F, Gallo RC, Croce CM (1982b). Chromosomal assignment of the human homologues of feline sarcoma virus and avian

myeloblastosis virus *onc* genes. Proc Natl Acad Sci USA
79:4714.

Der CJ, Krontiris TG, Cooper GM (1982). Transforming genes
of human bladder and lung carcinoma cell lines are
homologous to the *ras* genes of Harvey and Kirsten sarcoma
viruses. Proc Natl Acad Sci USA 79:3637.

D'Eustachio P, Pravtcheva D, Marcu K, Ruddle FH (1980).
Chromosomal location of the structural gene cluster
encoding murine immunoglobulin heavy chains. J Exp Med
151:1545.

Ellis RW, DeFeo D, Shih TY, Gonda MA, Young HA, Tsuchida N,
Lowy DR, Scolnick EM (1981). The p21 *src* genes of Harvey
and Kirsten sarcoma viruses originate from divergent
members of a family of normal vertebrate genes. Nature
292:506.

Fung Y-K T, Fadly AM, Crittenden LB, Kung H-J (1981). On
the mechanism of retrovirus-induced avian lymphoid
leukosis: deletion and integration of the proviruses.
Proc Natl Acad Sci USA 78:3418.

Hayward WS, Neel BG, Astrin SM (1981). Activation of a
cellular *onc* gene by promoter insertion in ALV-induced
lymphoid leukosis. Nature 290:475.

Hopkinson DA, Povey S, Solomon E, Bobrow M, Gormley IP
(1975). Confirmation of the assignment of the locus
determining ADA to chromosome 20 in man: data on
possible synteny of ADA and ITP in human-Chinese hamster
somatic cell hybrids. Cytogenet Cell Genet 16:159.

Kirsch IR, Morton CC, Nakahara K, Leder P (1982). Human
immunoglobulin heavy chain genes map to a region of
translocations in malignant B lymphocytes. Science
216:301.

Klein G (1981). The role of gene dosage and genetic transpositions in carcinogenesis. Nature 294:313.

Lalley PA, Minna JD, Francke U (1978). Conservation of
autosomal gene synteny groups in mouse and man. Nature
274:160.

Lenior GM, Preud'homme JL, Bernheim A, Berger R (1982).
Correlation between immunoglobulin light chain expression
and variant translocation in Burkitt's lymphoma. Nature
298:474.

Meera Khan P, Pearson PL, Wijnen LLL, Doppert BA,
Westerveld A, Bootsma D (1975). Assignment of inosine
triphosphatase gene to gorilla chromosome 13 and to
human chromosome 20 in primate-rodent somatic cell hybrids.
Cytogenet Cell Genet 16:420.

Noori-Daloii MR, Swift RA, Kung H-J (1981). Specific

integration of REV proviruses in avian bursal lymphomas. Nature 294:574.

Pall ML (1981). Gene-amplification model of carcinogenesis. Proc Natl Acad Sci USA 78:2465.

Parada LF, Tabin CJ, Shih C, Weinberg RA (1982). Human EJ bladder carcinoma oncogene is homologue of Harvey sarcoma virus *ras* gene. Nature 297:474.

Payne GS, Bishop JM, Varmus HE (1982). Multiple arrangements of viral DNA and an activated host oncogene in bursal lymphomas. Nature 295:209.

Roussel M, Saule S, Lagrou C, Rommens C, Beug H, Graf T, Stehelin D (1979). Three new types of viral oncogene of cellular origin specific for haematopoietic cell transformation. Nature 281:452.

Rowley JD, Testa JR (1982). Chromosome abnormalities in malignant hematologic diseases. Adv Cancer Res 36:103.

Sakaguchi AY, Naylor SL, Shows TB (1982). A sequence homologous to Rous sarcoma virus v-*src* is on human chromosome 20. Prog Nuc Acids Res Mol Biol in press.

Sheiness D, Bishop JM (1979). DNA and RNA from uninfected vertebrate cells contain nucleotide sequences related to the putative transforming gene of avian myelocytomatosis virus. J Virol 31:514.

Shilo B-Z, Weinberg RA (1981). DNA sequences homologous to vertebrate oncogenes are conserved in *Drosophila melanogaster*. Proc Natl Acad Sci USA 78:6789.

Shows TB, Sakaguchi AY, Naylor SL (1982). Mapping the human genome, cloned genes, DNA polymorphisms, and inherited disease. In Harris H, Hirschhorn K (eds): "Advances in Human Genetics," New York and London: Plenum Press, vol 12, p 341.

Southern EM (1975). Detection of specific sequences among DNA fragments separated by gel electrophoresis. J Mol Biol 98:503.

Spector DH, Varmus HE, Bishop JM (1978). Nucleotide sequences related to the transforming gene of avian sarcoma virus are present in DNA of uninfected vertebrates. Proc Natl Acad Sci USA 75:4102.

Stehelin D, Varmus HE, Bishop JM, Vogt PK (1976). DNA related to the transforming gene(s) of avian sarcoma viruses is present in normal avian DNA. Nature 260:170.

Swan D, D'Eustachio P, Leinwand L, Seidman J, Keithley D, Ruddle FH (1979). Chromosome assignment of the mouse κ light chain genes. Proc Natl Acad Sci USA 76:2735.

Swan DC, McBride OW, Robbins KC, Keithley DA, Reddy EP, Aaronson SA (1982). Chromosomal mapping of the simian sarcoma virus *onc* gene analogue in human cells. Proc Natl Acad Sci USA 79:4691.

Tischfield JA, Creagan RP, Nichols EA, Ruddle FH (1974). Assignment of a gene for adenosine deaminase to human chromosome 20. Hum Hered 24:1.

Weinberg RA (1982). Oncogenes of spontaneous and chemically induced tumors. Adv Cancer Res 36:149.

Weiss MC, Green H (1967). Human-mouse hybrid cell lines containing partial complements of human chromosomes and functioning human genes. Proc Natl Acad Sci USA 58:1104.

Zabel BU, Naylor SL, Sakaguchi AY, Shows TB, Gusella JF, Housman D, Shine J, Bell GI (1982). High resolution *in situ* hybridization: localization of a DNA restriction polymorphism, the human proopiomelanocortin gene, and the human insulin gene. Am J Hum Genet 34:153A.

Oncogenes and Retroviruses: Evaluation of Basic Findings and Clinical Potential, pages 105–118
© 1983 Alan R. Liss, Inc., 150 Fifth Avenue, New York, NY 10011

VIRAL SEQUENCES DETERMINING THE ONCOGENICITY OF AVIAN
LEUKOSIS VIRUSES

A.M. Skalka[1], P.N. Tsichlis[2], R. Malavarca[1], B.
Cullen[3], and G. Ju[3]

[1]Roche Institute of Molecular Biology, Nutley,
NJ; [2]Laboratory of Tumor Virus Genetics, National
Cancer Institute, Bethesda, MD; [3]Hoffmann-
La Roche Inc., Nutley, NJ

Exogenous and Endogenous Avian Leukosis Viruses (ALV)

Endogenous retroviruses are derived from proviral DNAs
which at some time in evolution become integrated in normal
germ-line cells of an organism and are thereafter transmitted
in a Mendelian fashion. The endogenous proviruses of
chickens represent a partially defined set of genetically-
related sequences. They are integrated at a number of loci
characterized by different levels of expression. Expression
from one of these loci, ev-2, gives rise to a replication-
competent virus called RAV-0 which has served as a prototype
of the endogenous ALV's (see Coffin, 1982 for review).

Although the genetic map and the overall structure of
the endogenous ALV's is similar to that of exogenous ALV's
acquired by horizontal infection, distinct biological
differences exist between the two. The genetic information
for these differences is located in the 3' end of the genome
and include: (1) The host range; a property defined by the
env gene which for endogenous viruses is always subgroup E
(Robinson, 1978); (2) The growth rate; exogenous viruses
tend to grow to higher titers in tissue culture (Tsichlis
and Coffin, 1980); and (3) The ability to cause disease;
all known exogenous ALV's are pathogenic for chickens,
causing a variety of neoplastic diseases with on-set
approximately 4-12 months after infection.

ALV RNA Genome:

	EXOGENOUS	ENDOGENOUS
Onset of disease:	4-12 mos.	—
Subgroup (host range):	A, B, C, D	E
Growth rate (virus titers):	High	Low
Diseases:	Lymphoma (B-cell) + others: eg. Sarcoma Carcinoma Osteopetrosis etc.	None

Table 1. Comparison of genome structure and biological properties of exogenous and endogenous ALVs. The genome map indicates the approximate location of the viral genes, gag, pol and env and the 5' and 3' regions which are encoded in the U5 and U3 regions of the LTRs of viral DNA. The wavy line at the 3' end represents the poly A tail on the viral RNA genomes.

This relatively slow development of disease is distinct from the rapid (7-21 day) on-set observed with the acute transforming viruses which transduce cellular oncogenes (Bishop & Varmus, 1982) and are not considered here.   In contrast to exogenous ALV's, the endogenous viruses are non-oncogenic in the chicken (Crittenden, et al, 1980; Robinson, et al, 1982).

Results derived from the isolation and biological analysis of a number of recombinant viruses with genetic contributions from both endogenous and exogenous ALV parents, provided evidence that the envelope gene does not specify oncogenicity (Robinson, et al, 1979). These same studies suggested that sequences downstream of env, believed to be important in control of viral RNA transcription, were critical. Among the recombinants analyzed, one (NTRE7) was of particular interest. Mapping data based on analysis of component proteins and RNA oligonucleotides showed it to be identical to RAV-0 with the exception of a region approxi-

mately 300-400 nucleotides from the 3' end which is derived
from its exogenous parent, the Prague B strain of RSV.
Despite the fact that most of its genome is from the RAV-0
endogenous parent, this recombinant exhibits two properties
characteristic of exogenous viruses: It grows to high titer
and is oncogenic. [The latter property is, however, modified
since the recombinant virus seems somewhat less virulent
than its exogenous parent and it generates a different
spectrum of neoplasia (Robinson, et al, 1982)].

    In order to identify the region responsible for these
properties, we have determined the nucleotide sequence of
NTRE7 and RAV-0 (Tsichlis, et al, 1982) and compared our
results with sequence data already available for the Prague
strain of ASV (Schwartz, et al, 1982). The sequences were
determined using molecular clones of covalently-closed
circular viral DNA obtained from NTRE7 or RAV-0 infected
cells. Thus, although the viral genome is RNA, the data are
expressed as DNA.

Sequence Comparison between NTRE7 and Its Exogenous
and Endogenous Parent

    Figure 1 shows results from analyses which include the
region from the end of the envelope gene, through a noncoding stretch and into the U3 and R regions of the LTR.
This corresponds to the 3' end of the viral RNA genome. Our
analyses extend into the U5 region of the LTR and a noncoding region both derived from the 5' end of the viral RNA.

    The comparison shows that the NTRE7 and RAV-0 sequences
are identical through the end of env. Following this is a
stretch of DNA which is quite similar in all three viruses,
although identity remains with RAV-0. This conserved region,
of about 130 nucleotides, occurs as a direct repeat (dr) on
either side of the src gene in non-defective Prague RSV
(Schwartz, et al, 1982). We believe that the recombination
event which generated NTRE7 occurred at the end of this
conserved region (-440 to -417), within 23 base pairs that
are identical in all 3 viral genomes. In the region distal
to this section NTRE7 is identical to its exogenous Prague
ALV parent. Interestingly, following the presumed crossover
point there is a region of about 148 base pairs that is
present in the Prague virus and NTRE7, but completely absent
in RAV-0. This region which we call XSR (exogenous specific
region) will be discussed again below.

```
          -670      -660      -650      -640      -630      -620      -610      -600
tdPrRSV  GGACTGCTTTTGGGGCTTGTAGTTATCTTATTGCTAGTAGTGTGCCTGCCTTGCCTTTTACAATTTGTGTCTAGTAGTAT

NTRE-7   TTGCTAGTAGTGTGCCTGCCTTGCCTTTTGCAAATTGTGTCCAGTAGCATCCGAAAGATGATTAATAATTCAATCAGCTA
         :::::::::::::::::::::::::::::::::::::::::::::::::::::::::::::::::::::::::::::::::::
RAV 0    TTGCTAGTAGTGTGCCTGCCTTGCCTTTTGCAAATTGTGTCCAGTAGCATCCGAAAGATGATTAATAATTCAATCAGCTA

          -590      -580      -570      -560      -550      -540      -530 env
tdPrRSV  TCGAAAGATGATTAATAGTTCAATCAACTATCATACTGAATACAGGAAGATGCAGGGCGGAGCAGTCTAGAGCTCAGTTA

NTRE-7   TCACACGGAATATAAGAAGTTGCAAAAGGCTTGTAGGCAGCCCGAAAATGGAGCAGTGTAAAGCAGTACATGGGTGGTGG
         :::::::::::::::::::::::::::::::::::::::::::::::::::::::::::::::::::: ::::::::::::::
RAV 0    TCACACGGAATATAAGAAGTTGCAAAAGGCTTGTAGGCAGCCCGAAAATGGAGCAGTGTAAAGCAGTACATGGGTGGTGG

          -510      -500      -490      -480      -470      -460      -450      -440
                                                              env
tdPrRSV  TAATAATCCTGCGAATCGGGCTGTAACGGGGCAAGGCTTGACTGAGGGGACCCATGATGTGTATAGGCGTCAAGCGGGGCT
         ::    ::   :::::::::::::::::::::::::::::::::::::::::          ::::::::::   :::::::
NTRE-7   TATGAAACTTGCGAATCGGGCTGTAACGGGGCAAGGCTTGACTGAGGGGACTACAGTATGTATAGGCGAAAGGCGGGGCT
         :::::::::::::::::::::::::::::::::::::::::::::::::::::::::::::::::::::::::::::::::::
RAV 0    TATGAAACTTGCGAATCGGGTTGTAACGGGGCAAGGCTTGACTGAGGGGACTACAGTATGTATAGGCGAAAGGCGGGGCT

          -430      -420      -410      -400      -390      -380      -370      -360
tdPrRSV  TCGGTTGTACGCGGATAGGAATCCCCTCAGGACAATTCTGCTTGGAATATGATGGCGTCTTCCCTGTTTTGCCCTTAGAC
         :::::::::::::::::::::::::::::::::::::::::::::::::::::::::::::::::::::::::::::::::::
NTRE-7   GCGGTTGTACGCGGATAGGAATCCCCTCAGGACAATTCTGCTTGGAATATGATGGCGTCTTCCCTGTTTTGCCCTTAGAC
         :::::::::::: ::::: ::::::::: :
RAV 0    TCGGTTGTACGCGGTTAGGAGTCCCCTCAGGATATA

          -350      -340      -330      -320      -310      -300      -290      -280
tdPrRSV  TATTCGAGTTGCCTCTGTGGATTAGGGCTGGAGGCAGCACGGATAGTCTGATGGCCAAATAAGGCAGGCAAGACAGCTAT
         :::::::::::::::::::::::::::::::::::::::::::::::::::::::::::::::::::::::::::::::::::
NTRE-7   TATTCAAGTTGCCTCTGTGGATTAGGGCTGGAGGCAGCACGGATAGTCTGATGGCCAAATAAGGCAGGCAAGACAGCTAT

RAV 0

          -270      -260      -250      -240      U3   -220      -210      -200
tdPrRSV  TTGTAACTGCGAAATACGCTTTTGCATAGGGGAGGGGGAAATGTAGTCTTATGCAATACTCCTGTAGTCTTGCAACATGCT
         :::::::::::::::::::::::::::::::::::::::::::::::::::::::::::::::::::::::::::::::::::
NTRE-7   TTGTAACTGCGAAATACGCTTTTGCATAGGGGAGGGGGAAATGTAGTCTTATGCAATACTCCTGTAGTCTTGCAACATGCT
                    ::::::::::::::::::::::::::::::::::::::::::::           ::: : ::
RAV 0    GTAGTTG          CGCTTTTGCATAGGGGAGGGGGAAATGTAGTCAAATAGAGCCAGAG        GCA CCTGAA

          -190      -180      -170      -160      -150      -140          -130      -120
tdPrRSV  TATGTAACGATGAGTTAGCAATATGCCTTACAAGGAAAGAAAAGGCACCGTGCA       TGCCGATTGGTGGTAGTAA
         ::::::::::::::::::::::::::::::::::::::::::::::::::::::::       ::::::::::::::::::::
NTRE-7   TATGTAACGATGAGTTAGCAATATGCCTTACAAGGAAAGAAAAGGCACCGTGCA       TGCCGATTGGTGGCAGTAA
                                ::  : :::::: ::::: ::          ::: ::::::::::
RAV 0    AAGTCTAAAGA          CCAAATAAGGA     AAAAG CAA GACATTC CATATGCTCATTGGTGGCGACTA

          -110      -100      -90       -80       -70       -60       -50       -40
tdPrRSV  GGTGGTACGATCGTGCCTTATTAGGAAGGTATCAGACGGGTCTAACATGGATTGGACGAACCACTGAATTCCGCATCGCA
         :::::::::::::::::::::::::::::::::::::::::::::::::::::::::::::::::::::::::::::::::::
NTRE-7   GGTGGTACGATCGTGCCTTATTAGGAAGGTATCAGACGGGTCTAACATGGATTGGACGAACCACTGAATTCCGCATCGCA
                                :::::::             : :::
RAV 0    GATAA          GGAAGGAATGACGCA     A GGACATATGGGCGTGAGACGAAGCTATGTACGA

          -30       -20       -10  U3      R    +10    R     U5  +30      +40
tdPrRSV  GAGATATTGTATTTAAGTGCCTAGCTCGATACAATAAAGCCATTTTACCATTCACCACATTGGTGTGCACCTGGGTTGA
         :::::::::::::::::::::::::::::::::::::::::::::::::::::::::::::::::::::::::::: ::::: ::
NTRE-7   GAGATATTGTATTTAAGTGCCTAGCTCGATACAATAAAGCCATTTTACCATTCACCACATTGGTGTGCACTTGGGTAGA
                 ::: ::::                   :::::::::::::::::::::::::::::::::::::::::::: :::
RAV 0    TTATATAAGCTGTTGCCACCATCAAATAAAGCCATTTTACCATTCACCACATTGGTGTGCACCTGGGTAGA

          +50       +60       +70       +80       +90    U5     +110      +120
tdPrRSV  TGGCCGGACCGTCGATTCCCTAACGATTGCGAACACCTGAATGAAGCAGAAGGCTTCATTTGGTGACCCCGACGTGATAG
         ::: :::::: ::::::::::::::::::::::::::::::::::::::::::::::::::::::::::::::::::::::::
NTRE-7   TGGACAGACCGTTGAGTCCCTAACGATTGCGAACACCTGAATGAAGCAGAAGGCTTCATTTGGTGACCCCGACGTGATCG
         :::::::::::::::::::::::::::::::::::::::::::::::::::::::::::::::::::::::::::::::::::
RAV 0    TGGACAGACCGTTGAGTCCCTAACGATTGCGAACACCTGAATGAAGCAGAAGGCTTCATTTGGTGACCCCGACGTGATCG
```

The identity of NTRE7 and the exogenous ALV parent
extends through the U3 region of the LTR. We had shown
earlier that the endogenous U3 region is markedly different
from that of exogenous viruses, whereas the R and U5 regions
are very similar (Hishinuma, et al, 1981). The data in
Figure 1 verify our earlier results.

Figure 2 is a diagramatic summary of the sequence
data. It illustrates that the recombination which generated
NTRE7 occurred distal to the <u>env</u> gene and shows that the U3
region of the LTR originates from the exogenous parent.
Since R is essentially the same in both parents and the
remainder of the DNA is derived from the 5' end of the

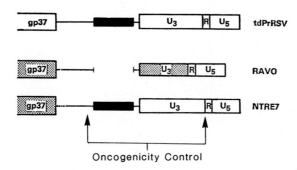

*Figure 2. Illustration of the genetic origin of NTRE7 from
its exogenous and endogenous ALV parents. Regions to the
left and right of the arrows are from RAV-0; between the
arrows from the tdPrRSV parent. The approximately 400 base
pair sequence which comprises the latter is presumed to
include the functions which specify oncogenicity. The
black rectangle represents the XSR.*

---

*Figure 1. Comparison of nucleotide sequences of the LTR
and adjacent regions of RAV-0 and NTRE7 with sequences
deduced for Prague td from the Prague ASV data of Schwartz,
et al, (1982). Lines indicate the limits of defined genetic
regions. Transcription control signals in the U3 region are
underlined. Homologies are indicated by dots; gaps have
been introduced to best align the sequences. The numbering
standard is from Schwartz, et al, (1982).*

virus, we conclude that the region which controls oncogenicity must lie within these 400 nucleotides including XSR and the U3 region of the LTR. In the following, we consider current information relevant to the XSR.

ASV ⟶ ALVs and the XSR

A comparison of sequence data for two strains of avian sarcoma viruses (ASVs), the Prague ASV, progenitor of the exogenous parent of NTRE7 and the independently isolated Schmidt-Ruppin ASV, shows that the XSR is found at different locations in the two transforming viruses (Figure 3). We conclude, therefore, that whatever function the XSR may encode, it cannot be dependent on genetic location. The transformation defective (td) viruses of both strains are presumed to arise by a homologous recombination between the 130 bp direct repeats (dr) which, as mentioned above, flank the src genes (Czernilowsky, et al, 1980). In the case of the Prague strain, the XSR is retained in the resulting td virus. With the Schmidt-Ruppin strain, however, we would expect the sequence to be lost with src since, like the oncogene, it lies between the dr sequences. Both Prague and Schmidt-Ruppin td's are oncogenic ALV's, although they differ in the spectrum of diseases they produce. It is possible, therefore, that the XSR plays some role in determining the oncogenic spectrum of a virus and further exploration of its function is certainly warranted. However, for the present it seems unlikely that this sequence is essential for oncogenicity per se.

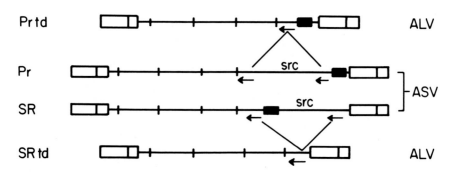

Figure 3. Presumed origin of ALV (td's) from ASV. The black rectangle represents the XSR. The open rectangles represent the LTRs; the wider section is U3, the narrower U5 and the line dividing them is R. The direct repeats

flanking the oncogene <u>src</u> are indicated by arrows; the boundaries of viral genes by vertical lines, Pr = Prague strain (sequence of Schwartz, et al, 1982); SR = Schmidt-Ruppin (sequence from Czernilowsky, et al, 1980).

The Viral LTRs

The remaining difference between the 3' ends of the genomes of RAV-0 and NTRE7 lies within the U3 region of the LTR. The viral LTR is presumed to function in at least two critical stages of viral replication. One is in integration of proviral DNA into the host chromosome, thought to involve an inverted repeat encoded in the left and right termini of the U3 and U5 regions respectively. The second is in control of transcription of the provirus. According to the "promoter insertion" model (Hayward, et al, 1981), in order to exert its influence on cellular oncogenes, ALV DNA must first integrate nearby. Although we cannot exclude the possibility that RAV-0 is not oncogenic because it cannot integrate near any cellular oncogenes, analyses to date have failed to reveal any specificity with respect to cellular integration sites (Lerner, et al, 1981). Thus for the present, or until more sensitive assays prove otherwise, it seems unlikely that integration-specificity distinguishes oncogenic from non-oncogenic ALV's.

Both endogenous and exogenous U3 regions contain sequences which resemble important eukaryotic transcription control signals. These include a TATA box (-30 to -24) which specifies the starting point of transcription (Gannon, et al, 1979) and a polyadenylation signal (-7 to -2) for termination; (after the CA at the right end of R; + 21. Konkel, Tilghman and Leder, 1978). The U3 regions of NTRE7 and RAV-0 differ most significantly to the left of the TATA box, where only short regions of homology can be assigned (see also Hishinuma, et al, 1981). It is this region, the approximately 200 base pairs upstream of the transcription initiation site, which is presumed to encode transcription promoter functions (McKnight and Kingsbury, 1982). Thus our results are consistent with the notion that promoter function might distinguish oncogenic from non-oncogenic viruses.

Transcription Studies in vivo

We have developed a sensitive biological assay to

measure transcription promoter activity from the avian ALV
LTR's (Cullen, et al, manuscript in preparation). The
basis for the assay, a modification of a system first
developed by Stacey and Hanafusa (1978), is illustrated
in Figure 4.

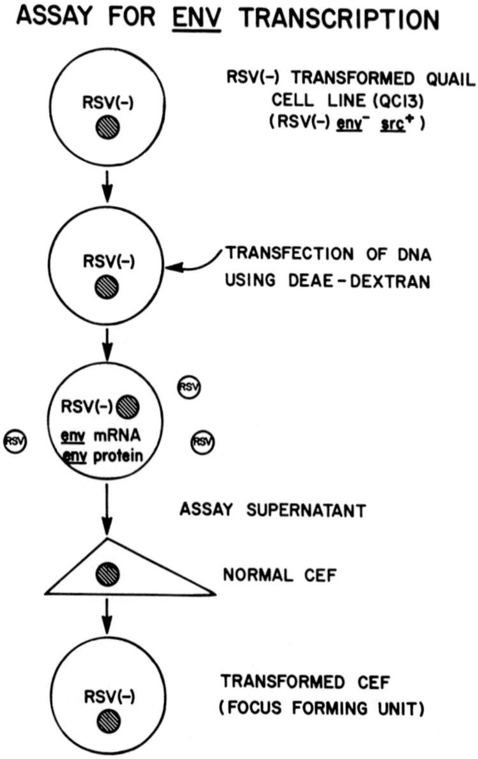

Figure 4. A complementation assay to measure transcription-
promoter activity. Steps are summarized in the text.

In it we utilize a quail cell line which has been transformed
with the Bryan high titer strain of RSV. The genome of
this virus contains src but lacks the env gene. Therefore,
although particles are produced by transformed cells they
are non-infectious because they lack the outer membrane
proteins which bind to specific receptors on sensitive
cells. The assay is based on complementation of this env

defect. Cells are exposed to test DNAs and at a defined
time thereafter, the number of infectious particles produced
is measured in a focus assay on sensitive chick embryo
fibroblasts. Stacey and Hanafusa (1978) showed earlier by
microinjection of env mRNA, that the number of infectious
transforming particles produced is proportional to the
amount of mRNA introduced. With Stacey we showed that
retroviral DNA clones containing the env gene are similarly
active, and that the DNA is transcribed almost immediately
after injection into the nucleus (Kopchick, et al, 1981).
In our modified transfection assays DNA is introduced using
the DEAE dextran technique, in amounts just saturating for
the focus assay response.

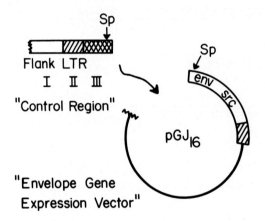

*Figure 5. Construction of plasmid clones with control
region cassettes. Restriction endonuclease sites used to
construct the clones and to manipulate individual regions
within the casettes are identified in Table 2. Sp = env
mRNA splice sites.*

Figure 5 shows a diagram of the cloned DNA used in our
analyses. The basic backbone of each clone tested is the
same; a plasmid derivative of pBR322 containing the 3' end
of ASV DNA including the env gene, the src gene and the
distal LTR to ensure correct termination of viral mRNA. We
utilize a convenient restriction site just in front of the
env RNA splice site to insert a variety of cassettes which
can control env gene expression. The cassettes, also
derived from cloned DNAs, have 3 components: I. Different
types of flanking regions upstream of the LTRs; II.

LTRs; and III. The 5' leader regions with a convenient restriction site beyond the required upstream <u>env</u> splice site.

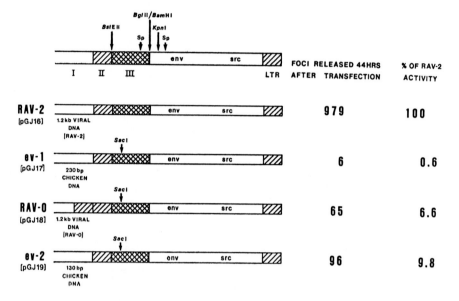

Table 2. Comparison of complementation activity with plasmid DNA clones containing different controlling casettes. The bold lettering at the left indicates the origin of the LTR (Region II) in each casette. The plasmid clone is identified in parenthesis below. The composition of flanking DNA (Region I) is also indicated. In each test quail CL3 cells in 33 mm plates were exposed to 500 ng of covalently cloned plasmid in the presence of 1 ug/ul DEAE dextran (in 0.2 ml) for 1/2 hour. Medium was then applied. Supernatants were sampled 44 hours later to assay for production of focus forming units on chick embryo fibroblasts as described earlier (Kopchick, et al, 1981).

Table 2 shows some results from our comparison of exogenous and endogenous LTRs. The exogenous virus RAV-2 and endogenous RAV-0 cassettes were both derived from circular premutations of cloned retroviral DNAs. Thus, the upstream flanking region in both cases comes from the 3' ends of the viral genomes. The RAV-2 cassette was most active, giving approximately 1,000 focus-forming units at a

standard collection time. For comparative purposes, this
value is set as 100%. Under the same conditions, the RAV-0
cassette was only about 7% as active.

In these tests an ev-2 cassette derived from the left
LTR of the integrated provirus is slightly more active than
RAV-0. Thus, the presence of 2 LTRs in the RAV-0 clone may
decrease the response somewhat. In the chicken chromosome
the LTR at the ev-2 locus is much less active than that of
integrated RAV-0 even though it is the locus from which
RAV-0 originates. This difference is probably due to
modifications of the ev-2 LTR which are not present on the
RAV-0 LTR (e.g. methylation, discussed by Scholl, et al,
1982). Such preferential modification would not be present
on our cloned DNAs which have been propagated in bacterial
cells. We have reported elsewhere (Scholl, et al, 1982)
that the nucleotide sequences of the ev-2 and RAV-0 LTRs
are identical.

The low activity with ev-1 was unexpected, since
sequence data show that the ev-2 and ev-1 LTR sequences are
almost identical (Scholl, et al, 1982). In other experiments
(not shown) we exchanged different components of the RAV-2
and ev-1 cassettes. We observed a 10 fold increase in
activity from the ev-1 cassette when it contained the
leader region (III) from RAV-2, whereas manipulation of the
flanking region (I) had no effect. We conclude from these
results that the ev-1 LTR is as active as a promotor as
that of RAV-0 but that ev-1 contains a defect in its leader
region. We are currently sequencing this region to determine
the nature of this defect.

Our findings indicate that the LTRs of ev 1, ev-2 and
RAV-0 have similar promoter activity, and that for all
three it is approximately 10 fold lower than that observed
with the LTR of exogenous virus RAV-2. This value is
similar to that obtained by others from analysis of the
number of transcripts in infected cells (Hayward. et al,
1980 and Baker, et al, 1981) and explains the differences
in growth rate which segregates with the U3 region of the
viruses (Tsichlis and Coffin, 1979).

Summary

Our analyses of the sequence of the recombinant virus
NTRE7 and comparison with its endogenous and exogenous ALV
parents indicate that a section of approximately 400 base
pairs at the 3' end of the genome encodes a function which
is required for oncogenicity. This section includes an
exogenous virus specific region (XSR) of approximately 148
base pairs and the U3 region of the LTR. At present it
seems most likely that the function required for oncogenicity
is the transcription promoter contained in the U3 region.

Assays designed to measure promoter activity of endogenous
and exogenous LTRs show a 10 fold difference between the
two. This result is consistent with the notion that RAV-0
is non-oncogenic because its promoter activity falls below
the limit required for oncogene activation. Our findings
suggest that there may be a critical threshold for oncogene
activation for which the RAV-2 value represents an upper
limit.

References

Baker B, Robinson H, Varmus HE, Bishop JM (1981). Analysis
  of endogenous avian retrovirus DNA and RNA: viral and
  cellular determinants of retrovirus gene expression.
  Virology 114:8.
Bishop JM and Varmus H (1982). Functions and origins of
  retroviral transforming genes. In Weiss R, Teich N,
  Varmus H, Coffin J (eds) "RNA Tumor Viruses". Cold Spring
  Harbor NY: Cold Spring Harbor Laboratory, p 999.
Coffin J (1982). Endogenous Viruses. In Weiss R, Teich N,
  Varmus H, Coffin J (eds) "RNA Tumor Viruses". Cold Spring
  Harbor NY: Cold Spring Harbor Laboratory, p 1109.
Crittenden LB, Hayward WS, Hanafusa H, Fadly AM (1980).
  Induction of neoplasms by subgroup E recombinants of
  exogenous and endogenous avian retroviruses. J Virol.
  33:915.
Cullen B, et al. Manuscript in preparation.
Czernilowsky AP, Levinson AD, Varmus HE, Bishop JM, Tischer
  E, Goodman HM (1980). Nucleotide sequence of an avian
  sarcoma virus oncogene (src) and proposed amino acid
  sequence for gene product. Nature 287:198.
Gannon F, O'Hare K, Perrin F, Le Penner JP, Benoist C,
  Cochet M, Breathnach MR, Royal A, Garapin A, Cami B,

Chambon P (1979). Organization and sequences at the 5' end of a cloned complete ovalbumin gene. Nature 278:428.

Hayward WS, Braverman SM, Astrin SM (1980). Transcriptional products and DNA structure of endogenous avian proviruses. Cold Spring Harbor NY: Cold Spring Harbor Symp Quant Biol 44:1111.

Hayward WS, Neel BG, Astrin SM (1981). Activation of a cellular onc gene by promoter insertion in ALV-induced lymphoid leukosis. Nature 290:475.

Hishinuma F, De Bona PJ, Astrin SM, Skalka AM (1981). Nucleotide sequence of acceptor site and termini of integrated avian endogenous provirus ev-1: integration creates a 6 bp repeat of host DNA. Cell 23:155.

Konkel DA, Tilghman SM, Leder P (1978). The sequence of the chromosomal mouse β-globin major gene: homologies in capping, splicing and poly (A) sites. Cell 15:1125.

Kopchick JJ, Ju G, Skalka AM, Stacey DW (1981). Biological activity of cloned retroviral DNA in microinjected cells. Proc Natl Acad Sci USA 78:4383.

Lerner TL, Skalka AM, Hanafusa H (1981). Integration of rous sarcoma virus DNA into chicken embryo fibroblasts: no preferred proviral acceptor site in the DNA of clones of singly infected chicken cells. J Virol 40:421.

McKnight SL, Kingsbury R (1982). Transcriptional control signals of a eucaryotic protein-coding gene. Science 217:316.

Robinson H (1978). Inheritance and expression of chicken genes which are related to avian sarcoma viruses. Cur Top Microbiol Immunol 83:1.

Robinson HL, Pearson MN, De Simone DW, Tsichlis PN, Coffin JM (1979). Subgroup-F avian leukosos-virus-associated disease in chickens. Cold Spring Harbor Symp Quant Biol 44:1133.

Robinson HL, Blais BM, Tsichlis PN, Coffin JM (1982). At least two regions of the viral genome determine the oncogenic potential of avian leukosis viruses. Proc Natl Acad Sci USA 79:1225.

Scholl DR, Kahn S, Malavarca R, Astrin S, Skalka AM (1982). Nucleotide sequence of the LTR and flanking cellular sequences of avian endogenous retrovirus ev-2: variation in RAV-0 expression cannot be explained by differences in primary sequence. J Virol (in press).

Schwartz D, Tizard R, Gilbert W (1982). The complete nucleotide sequence of the Pr-C strain of rous sarcoma virus. In Weiss R, Teich N, Varmus H, Coffin J (eds) "RNA Tumor Viruses". Cold Spring Harbor NY: Cold Spring

Harbor Laboratory, p 1340.

Stacey DW, Hanafusa H (1978). Nuclear conversion of micro-injected avian leukosis virion RNA into an envelope-glyco-protein messenger. Nature 273:779.

Tsichlis PN, Coffin JM (1979). Role of the c region in relative growth rates of endogenous and exogenous avian oncoviruses. Cold Spring Harbor Symp Quant Biol 44:1123.

Tsichlis PN, Coffin JM (1980). Recombinants between endogenous and exogenous avian tumor viruses: role of the c region and other portions of the genome in the control of replication and transformation. J Virol 33:238.

Tsichlis PN, Donehower L, Hager G, Zeller N, Malavarca R, Astrin S, Skalka AM (1982). Sequence comparison in the crossover region of an oncogenic avian retrovirus recom-binant and its non-oncogenic parent: genetic regions that control growth rate and oncogenic potential. Mol Cell Biol (in press).

Oncogenes and Retroviruses: Evaluation of Basic Findings
and Clinical Potential, pages 119–132
© 1983 Alan R. Liss, Inc., 150 Fifth Avenue, New York, NY 10011

THE ROLE OF HOST C-ONC GENES IN VIRAL AND NON-VIRAL NEOPLASIA

W. S. Hayward, B. G. Neel, C.-K. Shih, S. C.
Jhanwar and R. S. K. Chaganti
Memorial Sloan-Kettering Cancer Center
New York, NY 10021

More than fifteen different oncogenes have been identified in acute retroviruses isolated from avian and mammalian hosts (Coffin et al., 1981). These viral genes ("v-onc" genes) were derived from cellular genes ("c-onc" genes or "proto-oncogenes"), by recombination between host and viral sequences (Hanafusa, 1981; Bishop, 1981). The c-onc genes are present in all vertebrates (Bishop, 1981). The coding sequences of these genes have been highly conserved, suggesting that there is strong selective pressure to maintain their function in the host. Although the normal functions of the c-onc genes are not known, the phenotypes associated with expression of the v-onc genes suggest that they play some role in cell growth or differentiation.

As a consequence of the recombination event that generates an acute retrovirus, the onc gene is placed under the control of viral regulatory sequences. The v-onc gene is thus expressed at constitutive high levels in the infected cell, and does not respond to the regulatory signals that modulate expression of the corresponding c-onc gene. Changes within coding sequences may also accompany the conversion of a c-onc gene to a v-onc gene, but the possible contribution of these changes to the oncogenic potential of the v-onc genes has not been evaluated.

Recent studies have implicated the host c-onc genes more directly in a variety of neoplasms that are not

induced by viruses that carry oncogenes. The first such
system described was the B-cell lymphoma induced by avian
leukosis virus (ALV). ALV, which lacks an oncogene,
induces lymphomas by activating the c-myc gene (Hayward et
al., 1981), the cellular homolog of the oncogene (v-myc)
of MC29 virus (Mellon et al., 1978; Roussel et al.,
1979). More recently, several groups (Der et al., 1982;
Parada et al., 1982) have shown that "oncogenes" cloned
from human carcinoma cell lines are related to the c-ras
family of c-onc genes. The transforming capacity of these
genes, assayed by transfection of NIH/3T3 cells, appears
to correlate with the presence of a single point mutation
within the coding sequences of the human c-ras gene (R.
Weinberg, this symposium).

The possibility that chromosomal rearrangements might
also cause activation of c-onc genes has been suggested
(Hayward et al., 1981; Klein, 1981; Hayward et al.,
1982a). As discussed below, two c-onc genes have recently
been mapped to sites corresponding to breakpoints
associated with translocations in certain types of human
neoplasia. Thus, it seems likely that host c-onc genes
play a central role in a wide variety of neoplasms of both
viral and non-viral origin.

STRATEGIES FOR MYC GENE ACTIVATION: MC29 VIRUS VS ALV

MC29 is an acute retrovirus that causes rapid
transformation of tissue culture cells, and induces
neoplasms in infected animals after a relatively short
latent period (3-6 weeks) (Hanafusa, 1977; Graf and Beug,
1978; Moscovici and Gazzolo, 1982; Hayward et al.,
1982b). MC29 was derived by recombination between an
ALV-type virus and the cellular gene, c-myc, which has
become inserted in the viral genome, replacing the viral
pol gene and portions of gag and env. The myc gene is
thus controlled by viral regulatory sequences, and is
expressed at high levels in essentially all infected
cells. The v-myc gene product of MC29, a 110K gag-myc
fusion protein (Hayman, 1981; see Fig. 1), appears to lack
protein kinase activity (Bister et al., 1980; Sefton et
al., 1980). Recent evidence indicates that this protein
is a DNA binding protein, and is located primarily in the
nucleus (Abrams et al., 1982; Donner et al., 1982).

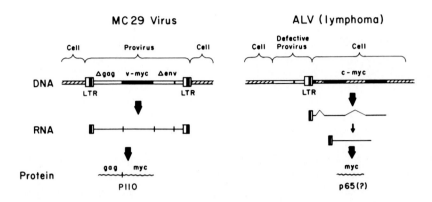

FIG. 1. Strategies of myc gene expression in ALV-and MC29 virus-induced tumors. The site of integration does not play a major role in transformation by MC29, since the oncogene (v-myc) is carried in the viral genome. Transformation by ALV, however, occurs only when the provirus is inserted adjacent to a c-onc gene. A defective ALV provirus is shown integrated in an orientation such that transcription of c-myc can initiate on the viral promoter, as found in most ALV-induced lymphomas. The myc gene product of MC29 is a gag-myc fusion protein. The putative product of the c-myc gene (p65) in ALV-induced lymphomas has not been isolated. DNA and RNA analyses (see text) indicate that it does not contain virus-encoded peptides. (From Hayward et al., 1982a.)

In contrast to MC29 virus, the avian leukosis viruses do not cause morphologic transformation of tissue culture cells at detectable frequency, and induce neoplasms in infected birds only after a latent period of 4-12 months (Graf and Beug, 1978; Hayward et al., 1982a). Induction of B-cell lymphoma by ALV is caused by activation of the host c-myc gene (Hayward et al., 1981). Transcriptional activation results from insertion of the viral regulatory sequences adjacent to the cellular gene (Neel et al., 1981; Payne et al., 1981; Hayward et al., 1981; Fung et al., 1981; Hayward et al., 1982a) (see Fig. 1). Since proviral integration is known to occur at many sites (Temin, 1980) - possibly at random - integrations that cause activation of c-myc are presumably rare.

The c-myc protein in ALV-induced lymphomas has not yet been identified. However, based on characterization of the c-myc DNA and mRNA in these tumors (Hayward et al., 1981; Neel et al., 1982a), it can be concluded that, unlike the gag-myc fusion proteins of MC29 virus, the myc protein in ALV-induced lymphomas does not contain virus-encoded peptides. The estimated size of this protein is 55-65,000 daltons (see Fig. 1).

In all of the ALV-induced lymphomas analyzed in detail, the provirus is defective, lacking the 5' LTR plus, in many cases, additional viral information (Neel et al., 1981; Payne et al., 1981; Fung et al., 1981; Rovigatti et al., 1982). The minimum amount of viral information found in these tumors is approximately 350 bases - roughly the size of the LTR (Fung et al., 1981; Rovigatti et al., 1982; H. Varmus, personal communication). Thus, it seems likely that all of the viral sequences required for c-myc activation are located within the LTR. The high incidence of defectiveness suggests that deletions play an essential role in c-myc activation. One explanation for this is that efficient transcription from the 3' LTR occurs only when the 5' LTR is absent. Since transcription of viral RNA (from the 5' LTR) proceeds into, and beyond, the initiation site within the 3' LTR (Hayward and Neel, 1981), normal transcription might block efficient utilization of the promoter in the 3' LTR.

STRUCTURE OF THE C-MYC GENE IN NORMAL AND IN ALV-TRANSFORMED TISSUES

DNA restriction fragments containing viral sequences, plus adjacent cellular sequences ("tumor junction fragments") were cloned from two independent ALV-induced lymphomas (Neel et al., 1982a), and compared with a c-myc clone from a normal chicken (see Fig. 2). Both of the tumor junction fragments contained c-myc sequences, in addition to the approximately 160 bases derived from the viral LTR.

The c-myc coding sequences in clones from both normal (Robins et al., 1982; Vennstrom et al., 1982; Neel et al.,

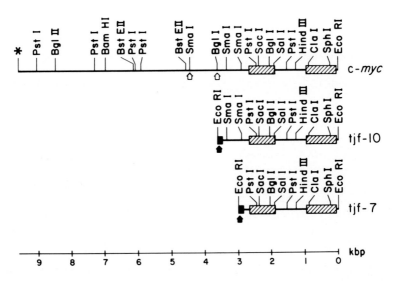

FIG. 2. Structure of the c-myc gene in normal cells and in ALV-induced lymphomas. DNA restriction fragments from two independent ALV-induced lymphomas were cloned into appropriate bacteriophage vectors, and selected by screening with an LTR probe. The normal c-myc clone, derived from a random library of normal chicken DNA, was selected by hybridization to a myc-specific probe. In all three clones, the myc-specific coding sequences were present in two exons (cross-hatched boxes), interrupted by a 1 kb intron. Viral LTR sequences (solid boxes) are covalently linked to the c-myc gene sequences in both tumor junction fragments (tjf7 and tjf10). Transcription in ALV-induced lymphomas generally initiates within the viral LTR (closed arrows). Possible cellular promoters for the normal c-myc gene (open arrows), were identified by transcription of the c-myc clone in a cell-free system (Neel, unpublished). (Adapted from Neel et al., 1982a).

1982a) and tumor tissues (Neel et al., 1982a) are encoded in two exons, interrupted by an intron of approximately 1 kb (Fig. 2). This contrasts with the structure of the v-myc gene of MC29, which lacks introns (see Fig. 1). The restriction maps of the two tumor junction fragments and the c-myc clone from normal cells were indistinguishable (see Fig. 2), with the exception that each of the junction

fragments had one additional EcoRI site, located within
the LTR of the integrated provirus. Thus, the c-myc genes
in the tumors had not sustained any substantial
rearrangements.

Transcription of c-myc in most ALV-induced lymphomas
initiates within the 3' LTR of the integrated provirus
(Fig. 2; closed arrows). In an effort to localize the
promoter for c-myc in normal cells, the c-myc clone was
used as a template in a cell-free transcription system (B.
G. Neel, unpublished). Two initiation sites, located
approximately 1 and 1.8 kb upstream from the 5' exon of
c-myc, were utilized in vitro (Fig. 2; open arrows). The
site of initiation in vivo has not been determined. A
minor c-myc transcript, approximately 4.2 kb in length,
can be identified in normal cells (unpublished
obervation). The size of this putative primary transcript
of c-myc is consistent with initiation from either of
these possible promoter sites in vivo, depending on where
the poly(A) addition signal is located.

A majority (26/30) of the ALV-induced lymphomas
analyzed in our studies (Neel et al., 1981; Rovigatti et
al., 1982) contained proviruses integrated downstream from
both potential promoters, but upstream from the 5' exon of
c-myc. In the remaining four tumors, the proviruses were
located further upstream, either between the two putative
promoters (1 tumor) or very close to the more distal
promoter (3 tumors). All of these proviruses were
inserted in the same transcriptional orientation as
c-myc. Thus, the viral promoter/regulator complex has, in
most cases, displaced the cellular promoter and regulatory
sequences.

Payne et al (1982) have identified one tumor in which
integration was downstream from c-myc, and several tumors
in which integration was upstream, but in the opposite
transcriptional orientation. Since the viral promoter
could not be utilized for c-myc activation in these
tumors, it seems likely that initiation occurs on a
cellular promoter. "Enhancer" sequences within the viral
LTR may exert some positive regulatory influence over
transcription, in a manner analogous to that demonstrated
for the 72 bp repeat of SV40 (Moreau et al., 1981; Gruss
et al., 1981). This, however, is apparently a less
efficient mechanism for activating c-myc, since more than

90% of tumors analyzed thus far contain proviruses integrated such that transcription could initiate on the viral promoter.

Cooper and Neiman (1981) have identified a second cellular gene - unrelated to c-myc and not linked to proviral sequences - that appears to be involved in lymphomagenesis. These authors have proposed a multi-step process in which the second gene acts at a late stage in tumor development. The mechanism responsible for activation of the second gene is unknown.

EXPRESSION OF C-MYC IN NORMAL TISSUES

The functions of the c-onc genes in normal cells is unknown. However, the fact that these genes are highly conserved in nature suggests that they play an essential role in the growth of the organism. Several examples of tissue-specific expression of c-onc genes have been reported (Chen, 1980; Gonda et al., 1982; Hayward et al., 1982b). These observations suggest a possible role in differentiation or growth control in specific stages of cell development.

We have analyzed the expression of c-myc in various avian tissues at different times after hatching (Hayward et al., 1982b; C.-K. Shih, unpublished). C-myc mRNA was detected in all tissues analyzed - generally at low levels (1-5 copies/cell). However, much higher levels were found in hematopoietic tissues (bursa, spleen, thymus, bone marrow) during the first 4 weeks after hatching, suggesting a possible role in early hematopoietic cell proliferation or differentiation. Several other lines of evidence are consistent with this idea: (i) higher levels of c-myc mRNA were found in isolated B and T cells (Gonda et al., 1982); (ii) c-myc is expressed at elevated levels in established cell lines representing early stages in B-cell development (Eva et al., 1982); (iii) c-myc (and also c-myb) are expressed at elevated levels in a promyelocytic leukemia cell line, HL60 (Westin et al., 1982a,b). Treatment of these cells with retinoic acid or other compounds induces terminal differentiation and a simultaneous shut off of c-myc and c-myb expression.

POSSIBLE INVOLVMENT OF C-ONC GENES IN HUMAN NEOPLASIA

Specific chromosomal abnormalities, especially translocations, are associated with many forms of human cancer (Rowley, 1980; Klein, 1981). The classic example is the 9,22 translocation that generates the Philadelphia chromosome associated with chronic myelogenous leukemia (CML) (Nowell and Hungerford, 1960). Specific chromosomal abnormalities have also been associated with Burkitt lymphoma (Manalov and Manalova, 1972; Mitelman, 1981), acute non-lymphoblastic leukemia (Rowley, 1980), and small cell carcinoma of the lung (Sandberg and Wake, 1981). One possible explanation for these specific chromosomal abnormalities in human cancers is that rearrangements place a strong transcriptional signal adjacent to the c-onc gene (Hayward et al., 1981; Klein, 1981).

To test this hypothesis, we have mapped several human c-onc genes, to determine whether they are located at chromosomal sites known to be involved in translocations associated with specific human malignancies (Neel et al., 1982b). Mapping was performed by in situ hybridization. With this technique it is possible not only to assign a gene to a specific chromosome, but also to determine the precise map location of the gene on the chromosome.

Two human c-onc genes, c-mos and c-myc, were localized to the long arm of chromosome 8 (Neel et al., 1982b). The human c-mos gene was mapped to band position 8q22, and the c-myc gene to position 8q24. These sites correspond to the breakpoints involved in specific translocations found in the M-2 subset of acute non-lymphoblastic leukemia (8q22), and Burkitt and other forms of non-Hodgkin's lymphoma (8q24).

It seems likely, therefore, that translocations of c-mos and/or c-myc are causally related to neoplastic disease. It is interesting that, in the Burkitt case, the translocation invariably involves chromosome 8 (position q24, the location of c-myc) plus one of three other chromosomes: 2, 14 or 22. These chromosomes carry the Ig κ, heavy, and λ chain Ig loci, respectively (Erikson et al., 1981; Kirsch et al., 1982; Malcolm et al., 1982). In two cases, these loci have been mapped precisely to the breakpoints involved in Burkitt lymphoma (Kirsch et al., 1982; Malcolm et al., 1982). The Ig loci are expressed at high levels in the target cells (early B-cells) involved in Burkitt lymphoma. Translocation of c-myc to an Ig locus, might, therefore, place c-myc under the control of the transcriptionally active Ig regulatory sequences.

CONCLUSIONS

Activation of the oncogenic potential of a c-onc gene can apparently result from two different types of genetic changes: alterations in regulatory sequences that affect the expression of the gene, and changes within the coding sequences that alter the properties of the gene product.

Activation of c-myc by ALV appears to be an example of a regulatory change, although the possibility that point mutations have occurred within the c-myc coding sequences cannot be excluded. It seems likely that Burkitt lymphoma, and other human neoplasms in which specific translocations occur, will also fall into this class of neoplasms resulting from regulatory changes in a normal c-onc gene. Two groups have demonstrated transformation of NIH/3T3 cells by c-onc genes (c-mos and c-ras) linked to LTR sequences (Oskarsson et al., 1980; Blair et al., 1981; DeFeo et al., 1981). Thus regulatory changes alone are sufficient to activate the oncogenic potential of these c-onc genes. In the acute transforming viruses, a c-onc gene has been placed under regulatory control of viral sequences located within the LTR. However, additional changes within the coding sequences (mutations or deletions) are also observed in some cases. The relative importance of these two factors has not yet been evaluated.

An apparent example of a change in coding sequences is the c-ras gene, implicated in various human carcinomas. A single base change within the coding region appears to be responsible for the ability of this gene to transform NIH/3T3 cells (R. Weinberg, this symposium).

The examples cited above include malignancies induced by a wide variety of carcinogenic agents, in hosts ranging from chicken to man. In each case, a genetic change (recombination, proviral integration, translocation, point mutation) affecting either regulatory or coding sequences, has altered the properties of a c-onc gene with profound consequences to the organism. Thus, a class of normal cellular genes (c-onc genes), first identified as oncogenes in acute retroviruses, appears to be the common denominator in malignancies of both viral and non-viral origin.

ACKNOWLEDGMENTS

We thank Anne Manwell and Ahamindra Jain for excellent technical assistance, and Lauren O'Connor for help in preparation of the manuscript. This work was supported by grant CA34502 from the National Institutes of Health, and by the Flora E. Griffin Memorial Fund. B.G.N. is a biomedical fellow in the Medical Scientist Training Program of the National Institutes of Health.

REFERENCES

Abrams HD, Rohrschneider LR, Eisenman RN (1982). Nuclear location of the putative transforming protein of avian myelocytomatosis virus. Cell 29:427.

Bishop JM (1981). Enemies within: The genesis of retrovirus oncogenes. Cell 23:5.

Bister K, Lee W-H, Duesberg PH (1980). Phosphorylation of the nonstructural proteins encoded by avian acute leukemia viruses and by avian Fujinami sarcoma virus. J Virol 26:617.

Blair DG, Oskarsson M, Wood TG, McClements WL, Fischinger PJ, Vande Woude GF (1981). Activation of the transforming potential of a normal cell sequence: A molecular model for oncogenesis. Science 212:941.

Chen J-H (1980). Expression of endogenous avian myeloblastosis virus information in different chicken cells. J Virol 36:162.

Coffin, JM, Varmus HE, Bishop JM, Essex M, Hardy WD, Martin GS, Rosenberg NE, Scolnick EM, Weinberg RA, Vogt PK (1981). A proposal for naming host cell-derived inserts in retrovirus genomes. J Virol 49:953.

Cooper GM, Neiman PE (1981). Two distinct candidate transforming genes of lymphoid leukosis virus induced neoplasms. Nature 292:857.

DeFeo D, Gonda MA, Young HA, Chang EH, Lowy DR, Scolnick EM, Ellis RW (1981). Analysis of two divergent rat genomic clones homologous to the transforming gene of

Harvey murine sarcoma virus. Proc Natl Acad Sci USA 78:3328.

Der CJ, Krontiris TG, Cooper GM (1982). Transforming genes of human bladder and lung carcinoma cell lines are homologous to the ras genes of Harvey and Kirsten sarcoma viruses. Proc Natl Acad Sci USA 79:3637.

Donner P, Greiser-Wilke I, Moelling K (1982). Nuclear localization and DNA binding of the transforming gene product of avian myelocytomatosis virus. Nature 296:262.

Erikson J, Martinis J, Croce CM (1981). Assignment of the genes for human imuunoglobulin chains to chromosome 22. Nature 294:173.

Eva A, Robbins KC, Andersen PR, Srinivasan A, Tronick SR, Reddy EP, Ellmore NW, Galen AT, Lautenberger JA, Papas TS, Westin EH, Wong-Staal F, Gallo RC, Aaronson SA (1982). Cellular genes analogous to retroviral onc genes are transcribed in human tumor cells. Nature, 295:116.

Fung Y-K, Fadly AM, Crittenden LB, Kung H-J (1981). On the mechanism of retrovirus-induced avian lymphoid leukosis: Deletion and integration of the proviruses. Proc Natl Acad Sci USA 78:3418.

Gonda TJ, Sheiness DK, Bishop JM (1982). Transcripts from the cellular homologs of retroviral oncogenes: distribution among chicken tissues. Mol Cell Biol 2:617.

Graf T, Beug H (1978). Avian leukemia viruses. Interaction with their target cells in vivo and in vitro. Biochem Biophys Acta Rev Cancer 516:269.

Gruss P, Dhar R, Khoury G (1981). Simian virus 40 tandem repeated sequences as an element of the early promoter. Proc Natl Acad Sci USA 78:943.

Hanafusa H. (1977). Cell transformation by RNA tumor viruses. In Fraenkel-Conrat, H and Wagner RR (eds): "Comprehensive Virology" Vol. 10, Plenum Press, NY, p401.

Hanafusa H (1981). Cellular origin of transforming genes of RNA tumor viruses. Harvey Lect 75:255.

Hayman MJ (1981). Transforming proteins of avian retroviruses. J Gen Virol 52:1.

Hayward WS, Neel BG (1981). Retroviral gene expression. Curr Top Microbiol Immunol 91:217.

Hayward WS, Neel BG, Astrin SM (1981). Activation of a cellular onc gene by promoter insertion in ALV-induced lymphoid leukosis. Nature 290:475.

Hayward WS, Neel, BG, Astrin SM (1982a). Avian leukosis viruses: Activation of cellular "oncogenes". In George Klein (ed): "Advances in Viral Oncology" Vol 1,

Raven Press, NY, p207.

Hayward WS, Shih C-K, Moscovici C (1982b). Induction of bursal lymphoma by myelocytomatosis virus-29 (MC29). In "Cetus-UCLA Symposium on Tumor Viruses and Differentiation" Liss, NY (in press).

Kirsch, IR, Morton, C, Nakahara, K, Leder P (1982). Human immunoglobulin heavy chain genes map to a region of translocations in malignant B lymphocytes. Science 216:301.

Klein G, (1981). Changes in gene dosage and gene expression: a common denominator in the tumorigenic action of viral oncogenes and non-random chromosomal changes. Nature 294:313.

Malcolm S, Barton P, Murphy C, Ferguson-Smith MA, Bently DC, Rabbits TH (1982). Localization of human immunoglobulin κ light chain variable region genes to the short arm of chromosome 2 by in situ hybridization. Proc. Natl. Acad Sci USA 79:4957.

Manalov G, Manalova Y (1972). Marker band in one chromosome 14 from Burkitt lymphomas. Nature 237:33.

Mellon P, Pawson A, Bister K, Martin GS, Duesberg PH (1978). Specific RNA sequences and gene products of MC29 virus. Proc Natl Acad Sci USA 75:5874.

Mitelman F (1981). Marker chromosome 14q+ in human cancer and leukemia. Advances in Cancer Research 34:141.

Moreau P, Hen R, Wasylyk B, Everett R, Gaub MP, Chambon P (1981). The SV40 72 base pair repeat has a striking effect on gene expression both in SV40 and other chimeric recombinants. Nucleic Acids Res 9:6047.

Moscovici C, Gazzolo L (1982). Transformation of hemopoietic cells with avian leukemia viruses. In Klein G (ed) "Advances in Viral Oncology" Vol 1 Raven Press, NY p83.

Neel BG, Gasic GP, Rogler CE, Skalka AM, Papas T, Astrin SM, Hayward WS (1982a). Molecular cloning of virus-cell junctions from ALV-induced lymphomas: Comparison with the normal c-myc gene. J Virol 44:158.

Neel BG, Hayward WS, Robinson HL, Fang J, Astrin SM (1981). Avian leukosis virus-induced tumors have common proviral integration sites and synthesize discrete new RNAs: Oncogenesis by promoter insertion. Cell 23:323.

Neel BG, Jhanwar SC, Chaganti RSK, Hayward WS (1982b). Two human c-onc genes are located on the long arm of chromosome 8. Proc Natl Acad Sci USA (in press).

Nowell PC, Hungerford DA (1960). A minute chromosome in human chronic granulocytic leukemia. Science 132:1497.

Oskarsson M, McClements WL, Blair DG, Maizel JV, Vande Woude GF (1980). Properties of a normal mouse cell DNA sequence (sarc) homologous to the src sequence of Moloney sarcoma virus. Science 207:1222.

Parada LF, Tabin CJ, Shih C, Weinberg RA (1982). Human EJ bladder carcinoma oncogene is homologue of Harvey sarcoma virus ras gene. Nature 297:474.

Payne GS, Bishop JM, Varmus HE (1982). Multiple arrangements of viral DNA and an activated host oncogene (c-myc) in bursal lymphomas. Nature 295:209.

Payne GS, Courtneidge SA, Crittenden LB, Fadly AM, Bishop JM, Varmus HE (1981). Analyses of avian leukosis virus DNA and RNA in bursal tumors: viral gene expression is not required for maintenance of the tumor state. Cell 23:311.

Robins T, Bister K, Garon C, Papas T, Duesberg P (1982). Structural Relationship between a normal chicken DNA locus and the transforming gene of the avian acute leukemia virus MC29. J Virol 41:635.

Roussel M, Saule S, Lagrou C, Rommens C, Beug H, Graf T, Stehelin D (1979). Three new types of viral oncogene of cellular origin specific for haematopoietic cell transformation. Nature 281:452.

Rovigatti UG, Rogler CE, Neel BG, Hayward WS, Astrin SM (1982). Expression of endogenous oncogenes in tumor cells. In "Fourth Annual Bristol-Myers Symposium on Cancer Research" Academic Press, NY p319.

Rowley JD (1980). Chromosome abnormalities in human leukemia. Annu Rev Genet 14:17.

Sanberg AA, Wake NN (1981). in Arrighi FE, Rao PN & Stubblefield E (eds): "Genes, Chromosomes, and Neoplasia" Raven Press, NY p297.

Sefton BM, Hunter T, Beemon K, Eckhart W (1980). Evidence that phosphorylation of tyrosine is essential for cellular transformation by Rous sarcoma virus. Cell 20:807.

Temin HM (1980). Origin of retroviruses from cellular moveable genetic elements. Cell 21:599.

Vennstrom B, Sheiness D, Zabielski J, Bishop JM (1982). Isolation and characterization of c-myc, a cellular homolog of the oncogene (v-myc) of avian myelocytomatosis virus strain 29. J Virol 42:773.

Westin EH, Gallo RC, Arya SK, Eva A, Souza LM, Baluda MA, Aaronson SA, Wong-Staal F (1982a). Differential expression of the amv gene in human hematopoietic cells. Proc Natl Acad Sci USA 79:2194.

Westin EH, Wong-Staal F, Gelman EP, Dalla-Favera RD, Papas
   TS, Lautenberger JA, Eva A, Reddy EP, Tronick SR,
   Aaronson SA, Gallo RC (1982b). Expression of cellular
   homologues of retroviral onc genes in human hematopoietic
   cells. Proc Natl Acad Sci USA 79:2490.

PROTEIN PRODUCTS OF ONC GENES

Oncogenes and Retroviruses: Evaluation of Basic Findings
and Clinical Potential, pages 135–147
© 1983 Alan R. Liss, Inc., 150 Fifth Avenue, New York, NY 10011

THE ASSOCIATION OF THE TRANSFORMING PROTEIN OF ROUS
SARCOMA VIRUS WITH TWO CELLULAR PHOSPHOPROTEINS

Joan S. Brugge, Diane Darrow, Leah A. Lipsich,
Wes Yonemoto

Department of Microbiology
State University of New York at Stony Brook
Stony Brook, New York   11794

INTRODUCTION

Oncogenic transformation by Rous sarcoma virus is
mediated by a single protein encoded by the viral gene
designated src (review, Bishop, Varmus 1982). Genetic
studies have indicated that this gene product, termed
$pp60^{src}$, is responsible for the initiation and maintenance of the pleiotrophic alterations in cellular
physiology and growth control which accompany RSV-induced
transformation (review). The precise mechanism whereby
$pp60^{src}$ elicits these diverse changes in cellular
metabolism is unknown; however, the analysis of mutant
viruses containing conditional and nonconditional
mutations in the src gene have provided evidence that
these pleiotrophic changes might result from the direct
interaction of $pp60^{src}$ with different cellular targets
(Weber, Friis 1979; Anderson, Beckman, Harms, Nakamura,
Weber 1981). In order to understand the mechanism of
RSV-induced transformation, it is important to understand
the molecular nature of these interactions between
$pp60^{src}$ and cellular proteins.

The $pp60^{src}$ protein was first identified by immunoprecipitation of cell lysates with serum (TBR) from
animals bearing RSV-induced tumors (Brugge, Erikson 1977)
and by translation of purified viral RNA in a reticulocyte cell-free lysate (Purchio, Erikson, Brugge, Erikson
1978). The $pp60^{src}$ protein has been shown to be

associated with a phosphotransferase activity specific for tyrosine residues (Collett, Erikson 1978; Levinson, Oppermann, Levintow, Varmus, Bishop 1978; Hunter, Sefton 1980). This activity is believed to be intrinsic to the protein since the pp60^{src} protein which has been produced in bacteria by introduction of a plasmid carrying the src gene possesses tyrosine-specific protein kinase activity (Gilmer, Erikson 1981; McGrath, Levinson 1982). Tyrosine phosphorylation is rare in eukaryotic cells and trans-formation by RSV causes a 7-10 fold increase in phos-phorylation of tyrosine in cellular proteins (Sefton, Hunter 1980). These results suggest that tyrosyl-phosphorylation is involved in pp60^{src}-mediated transfor-mation.

This manuscript will describe investigations of one aspect of the events which occur after RSV-induced transformation of chicken cells. These studies have focused on the interaction between pp60^{src} and two cellular phosphoproteins of M_r 90,000 (pp90) and 50,000 (pp50) which are associated in a protein complex with pp60^{src} in RSV-transformed cells (Hunter, Sefton 1980; Brugge, Erikson, Erikson 1981; Oppermann, Levinson, Levintow, Varmus, Bishop 1981). This protein complex was first identified by sedimentation analysis of RSV-transformed cell lysates on glycerol gradients (Brugge, Erikson, Erikson 1981). Two forms of pp60^{src} were resolved by immunoprecipitation with serum (TBR) obtained from rabbits bearing RSV-induced tumors (Fig. 1). The major portion of pp60^{src} sedimented as a monomer with a peak in fraction 20. However, a minor portion (approximately 1-5%) of pp60^{src} sedimented more rapidly. pp90 and pp50 were found to coprecipitate and cosediment with this minor fraction of pp60^{src}. These results suggest that a small portion of pp60^{src} is associated with pp90 and pp50. We have recently confirmed the trimolecular nature of this complex by immuno-precipitation of pp60^{src} and pp50 with monoclonal antibody directed against pp90 (Brugge, Yonemoto, Darrow, in press) and analogously, by immunoprecipitation of pp50 and pp90 with monoclonal antibody to pp60^{src} (Lipsich, Lewis, Brugge, unpublished results).

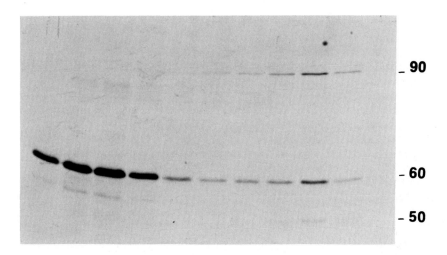

Fig. 1. Sedimentation analysis of ^{35}S-methionine-labeled
lysates from RSV-transformed chicken cells. Cells
transformed by the Schmidt-Ruppin (SR) strain of RSV
(subgroup A) were labeled for 24 hours with ^{35}S-
methionine, lysed in RIPA buffer and the lysate subjected
to sedimentation analysis as described (Brugge, Erikson,
Erikson 1981). Briefly, the cell lysate was clarified at
50,000 Xg and sedimented on a glycerol gradient in an SW
50.1 rotor for 17 hours at 49,000 RPM. The gradient
fractions were collected, incubated with TBR serum
preadsorbed with viral structural proteins, and the
immunoprecipitated proteins were analyzed on SDS-
polyacrylamide gels. Fractions 4-26 are shown here.
Sedimentation is from left to right.

The transforming proteins encoded by two distinct
avian sarcoma viruses (Fujinami and Yamaguchi 73 sarcoma
viruses) were also found to be a associated with pp90 and
pp50 (Lipsich, Cutt, Brugge 1982). Although the transforming genes from Rous, Fujinami and Yamaguchi 73
sarcoma viruses were derived from unique cellular genes
(review, Bishop, Varmus 1982) the proteins encoded by
these genes share considerable amino acid homology and
all three proteins have an associated tyrosine-specific

protein kinase activity (Kitamura, Kitamura, Toyoshima, Hirayama, Yoshida 1982; Shibuya and Hanafusa, personal communication). This suggests that pp90 and pp50 may play a common role in the events involved in transformation by avian sarcoma viruses which encode tyrosine-specific protein kinases.

In order to elucidate the functional role of this complex we have pursued several different investigations of this interaction between pp50, pp60^{src} and pp90. First, we have compared the expression of pp90 and pp50 in uninfected chicken cells to that found in ASV-transformed cells in order to determine whether the synthesis or phosphorylation of pp90 and pp50 is altered after RSV-induced transformation. Secondly, we have investigated the turnover and localization of the pp50:pp60^{src}:pp90 complex in ASV-transformed chicken cells.

Characterization of pp90 and pp50

We have found that pp90 is a relatively abundant protein in uninfected chicken cells, representing approximately 0.5-1 % of the total cell protein (Brugge, Erikson, Erikson 1981). pp90 is a phosphoprotein which contains several phosphorylated tryptic peptides, all of which contain phosphoserine. No detectable differences were observed in the phosphorylation of pp90 which is associated with pp60^{src} and pp50 (Hunter, Sefton 1980; Brugge, Erikson, Erikson 1981). Monoclonal antibody-directed against pp90 has been prepared and used to investigate the cellular distribution of pp90. pp90 was found to be associated with soluble cellular material when cells are fractionated by homogenization in hypotonic buffers or by extraction of cells with non-ionic detergent (Brugge, Yonemoto, Darrow 1982; Brugge, Yonemoto, Lipsich, Darrow 1982). Attempts to localize pp90 by immunohistochemical techniques have not revealed the association of pp90 with any specific cellular structures.

Oppermann, Levinson and Bishop (1981) have found that pp90 is identical to one of several proteins whose synthesis increases after incubation of cells at elevated temperatures (heat shock) or other "stress-inducing" conditions. Since the function of these "stress" proteins has not been identified it is premature to make correlations between this stress effect and viral transformation.

pp50 was detected in uninfected cells by comparison of the total cellular phosphoproteins from uninfected and RSV-transformed chicken embryo fibroblasts (Brugge, Darrow 1982; Gilmore, Radke, Martin 1982). Uninfected cells contain a single phosphorylated species of pp50 which contains phosphoserine. Transformed cells contain two species of pp50, one of which comigrates with pp50 from uninfected cells and an additional species which contains phosphotyrosine as well as phosphoserine. This latter species of pp50 is identical to the pp50 protein which is bound to pp60^{src} in RSV-transformed cell lysates. The presence of phosphotyrosine on a protein which is intimately associated with pp60^{src} suggests that pp50 may be a substrate of pp60^{src}-mediated phosphorylation.

Fractionation of cells into soluble and particulate fractions by homogenization of cells preincubated in hypotonic buffers indicated that pp50, like pp90, is a highly soluble cellular protein (Gates, Brugge, unpublished results).

The isolation of monoclonal antibody to pp90 has allowed us to determine whether pp50 is associated with pp90 in uninfected chicken cells. Figure 2 shows immunoprecipitation of ^{32}P-labeled uninfected and RSV-transformed chicken cell lysates. The antibody to pp90 immunoprecipitated a protein from uninfected cells (lane 1) which comigrated with the pp50 protein immuno-precipitated from RSV-transformed cell with either TBR serum (lane 3) or anti-pp90 (lane 4). The pp50 protein immunoprecipitated from normal chicken cell lysates with anti-pp90 (lane 1) was compared to the pp60^{src}-associated pp50 protein (from lane 3) by partial proteolytic cleavage with chymotrypsin (lanes 5 and 6). This analysis revealed that two of the phosphopeptides of the pp50 proteins were identical and the pp60^{src}-associated pp50 protein contained two additional phosphopeptides (designated with stars). These two phosphopeptides have

previously been shown to be specific to the phospho-
tyrosine-containing species of pp50. These results
suggest that pp50 is associated with pp90 in the absence
of pp60^{src} and that this pp90-bound species of pp50 does
not contain phosphotyrosine in uninfected chicken cells.

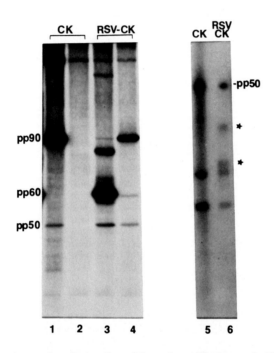

Fig. 2. Association of pp90 and pp50 in uninfected
chicken cells. Normal chicken cells (lanes 1 and 2) or
RSV-transformed chicken cells (lane 3 and 4) were labeled
with ^{32}P-orthophosphate for four hours. Cell lysates
were prepared and immunoprecipitated with monoclonal
antibody to pp90 (lanes 1 and 4), normal rabbit serum
(lane 2), or TBR serum (lane 3). The immunoprecipitated
proteins were prepared for electrophoresis on 7.5%
SDS-polyacrylamide gels as described previously (Brugge,
Erikson 1977).

Turnover and Localization of the pp50:pp60^{src}:pp90
Complex in RSV-transformed Cells

Figure 1 demonstrated that only a small proportion
of pp60^{src} is associated with pp50 and pp90 under
steady-state labeling conditions. In order to
investigate whether this complex-bound form of pp60^{src}
represented a small population of src molecules which
were stably associated with pp50 and pp90 or a constantly
cycling population of pp60^{src} molecules we performed the
following experiment. RSV-transformed cell lysates were
labeled with ^{35}S-methionine for 15 minutes and either
harvested immediately or chased for 30 minutes or 180
minutes with excess cold methionine. Cell lysates were
prepared and subjected to sedimentation analysis similar
to that shown in Figure 1. The results in Figure 3
demonstrate that most of newly synthesized molecules of
pp60^{src} are associated with pp50 and pp90. Within 30
minutes after removal of ^{35}S-methionine, two-thirds of
the previously bound molecules of pp60^{src} sedimented as a
monomer. After 180 minutes at least 90 percent of the
radiolabeled pp60^{src} sedimented as a monomer. These
results suggest that newly synthesized pp60^{src} molecules
bind preferentially to pp50 and pp90 and this interaction
is short-lived.

It has been shown previously that pp60^{src} is
synthesized on free polysomes and then associates with
the plasma membrane (Purchio, Jonanovich, Erikson 1981;
Lee, Varmus, Bishop 1979; Courtneidge, Levinson, Bishop
1980; Krueger, Wang, Goldberg 1980). It was therefore of
interest to determine whether pp50 and pp90 binds to
soluble or membrane bound form of pp60^{src}. ^{32}P-labeled
RSV-transformed cells were fractionated by homogenization
in hypotonic buffer. Soluble and particulate cellular
material were separated by sedimentation at 50,000 Xg.
After solubilization of the particulate material, the two
fractions were incubated with TBR serum or monoclonal
antibody to pp90. Figure 4 demonstrates that the
majority of pp60^{src} molecules fractionated with the
particulate cellular material. In contrast, pp50 and
pp90 were found associated with pp60^{src} molecules which
fractionated with soluble cellular material. Free pp90
also fractionated with the soluble cell material.

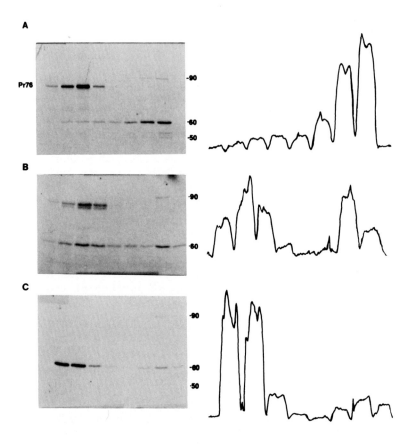

Fig. 3. Sedimentation analysis of cells pulse-labeled
with ^{35}S-methionine with and without a chase period in
the absence of ^{35}S-methionine. Cells transformed by the
SR-A strain of RSV were labeled for 15 minutes with
^{35}S-methionine (200 μc/ml) and either harvested directly
(A) or the medium was removed and replaced with standard
media plus 5X cold methionine and incubated for 30
minutes (B) or 180 minutes (C). Cell lysates were
prepared, subjected to sedimentation analysis, the
immunoprecipitated proteins were analyzed as described in
Figure 1.

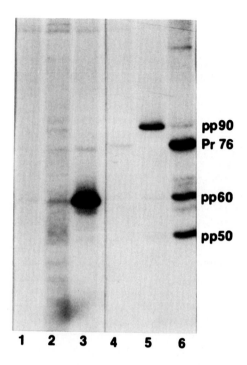

pp90
Pr 76

pp60

pp50

1 2 3 4 5 6

Fig. 4. Fractionation analysis of ^{32}P-labeled
RSV-transformed chicken cells. Cells transformed by the
SR-A strain of RSV were labeled for four hours with ^{32}P
(1 mc/ml). Cells were fractionated into soluble and
particulate fractions by a modification of the procedure
of Krueger and coworkers, as described by Brugge,
Yonemoto and Darrow (in press). Described briefly, the
cells were mechanically disrupted by homogenization in a
hypotonic buffer and fractionated by centrifugation at
50,000 Xg for 30 minutes. The supernatant was removed
and designated as the S50 fraction. The pellet was then
resuspended in a hypertonic buffer containing nonionic
detergent, and sedimented at 50,000 x g for 10 minutes.
The supernatant from this solubilized material was
designated, P50. Both the S50 and P50 fractions were
diluted with an equal volume of RIPA and immunoprecipitated as described.

Model to Describe the Interaction of $pp60^{src}$ with pp90 and pp50

The above results provide evidence to support the model described below of the events which occur shortly after the synthesis of $pp60^{src}$.

1) Newly synthesized molecules of $pp60^{src}$ which are phosphorylated on serine bind to pp90 and pp50. We have shown previously (Brugge, Erikson, Erikson 1981) that molecules of $pp60^{src}$ which are associated with pp90 and pp50 are phosphorylated on serine but contain less than 1% the content of phospho-tyrosine that is found in the free-unbound form of $pp60^{src}$. The results shown in Figure 2 suggest that pp50 and pp90 may be associated with each other before the binding of $pp60^{src}$. It is also of interest that $pp60^{src}$ is inactive as a protein kinase when bound to pp50 and pp90 (Brugge, Erikson, Erikson 1981).

2) After its association with $pp60^{src}$, pp50 is phosphorylated on tyrosine. The significance of this phosphorylation event in the functional role of this complex (Gates and Brugge, unpublished results) is uncertain since we and others (Oppermann, Levinson, Levintow, Varmus, Bishop, Kawai 1981) have found that pp50 is not phosphorylated in transformed mammalian cells. In addition we have recently found that pp50 is not phosphorylated in cells infected with a mutant virus (CH119 Lipsich, Brugge, Bryant and Parsons, unpublished results) which displays a temperature-dependent transformed phenotype. Despite the apparently normal binding of $pp60^{src}$ to pp50 and pp90, pp50 is not phosphorylated at the permissive temperature.

At some point either before or shortly after the association of $pp60^{src}$ with the membrane, the complex dissociates and $pp60^{src}$ is phosphorylated on tyrosine. The precise sequence of events which occur during and after the dissociation of this complex is not clear. Mutants of the Schmidt-Ruppin strain of RSV which contain temperature-sensitive defects in the src gene appear to be defective in the dissociation of the $pp50:pp60^{src}:pp90$ complex. Sedimentation analysis of mutant-virus infected cells at the nonpermissive temperature indicated that the majority of pp60^{src} molecules are associated with pp90 and pp50 (Brugge, Erikson, Erikson 1981).

This temporal sequence of events which occur after the synthesis of pp60^{src} suggests that pp90 and pp50 may be involved in processing events which take place before pp60^{src} reaches the plasma membrane. The functional nature of these events is not clear, however, the following possible roles are under consideration:

1) transport of pp60^{src} to the plasma membrane,
2) maintenance of the solubility of pp60^{src}, or
3) regulation of the phosphotransferase activity of pp60^{src}.

This work was supported by grant #CA27951 from the National Cancer Institute.

Anderson DD, Beckmann RP, Harms EH, Nakamura K, Weber MJ (1981). Biological properties of "partial" trans-formation mutants of Rous sarcoma virus and characterization of their pp60^{src} kinase. J Virol 37:445.

Bishop J, Varmus H (1982). Functions and origins of retroviral transforming genes. In Weiss, Teich, Varmus, Coffin (ed): "RNA Tumor Viruses. Cold Spring Harbor Press, p 999.

Brugge JS, Erikson RL (1977). Identification of a transformation-specific antigen induced by an avian sarcoma virus. Nature 269:346.

Brugge JS, Erikson E, Erikson RL (1981). The specific interaction of the Rous sarcoma virus transforming protein, pp60^{src}, with two proteins from chicken cells. Cell 25:363.

Brugge JS, Yonemoto W, Darrow D (1982). Interaction between the Rous sarcoma virus transforming protein and two cellular phosphoproteins: Analysis of the turnover and distribution of this complex. Mol Cell Biol, in press.

Brugge JS, Yonemoto W, Lipsich L, Darrow D (1982). Analysis of a protein complex involving pp60^{src} and two cellular phosphoproteins of M$_r$ 90,000 and 50,000. CETUS-UCLA Symposium on Tumor Viruses and Differentiation. In press.

Brugge JS, Darrow D (1982). Rous sarcoma virus-induced phosphorylation of a 50,000 molecular weight cellular protein. Nature 295:250.

Collett MS, Erikson RL (1978). Protein kinase activity associated with the avian sarcoma virus src gene product. Proc Natl Acad Sci USA 75:2021.

Courtneidge SA, Levinson AD, Bishop JM (1980). The protein encoded by the transforming gene of avian sarcoma virus (pp60^{src}) and a homologous protein in normal cells (pp60$^{proto-src}$) are associated with the plasma membrane. Proc Natl Acad Sci USA 77:3783.

Gilmer T, Erikson RL (1981). Rous sarcoma virus transforming protein, pp60^{src}, expressed in E. coli, functions as a protein kinase. Nature 294:771.

Gilmore T, Radke K, Martin GS (1982). Tyrosine phosphorylation of a 50K cellular polypeptide associated with the Rous sarcoma virus-transforming protein, pp60^{src}. Mol Cell Biol 2:199.

Hunter T, Sefton B (1980). Trasnforming gene product of Rous sarcoma virus phosphorylates tyrosine. Proc Natl Acad Sci USA 77:1311.

Kitamura N, Kitamura A, Toyoshima K, Hirayama Y, Yoshida M (1982) Avian sarcoma virus Y73 genome sequence and structural similarity of its transforming gene product to that of Rous sarcoma virus. Nature 297:205.

Krueger JG, Wang E, Goldberg AR (1980). Evidence that the src gene product of Rous sarcoma virus is membrane associated. Virology 101:25.

Lee JS, Varmus HE, Bishop JM (1979). Virus-specific messenger RNAs in permissive cells infected by avian sarcoma virus. J Biol Cehm 254:8015.

Levinson AD, Oppermann H, Levintow L, Varmus HE, Bishop JB (1978) Evidence that the transforming gene of avian sarcoma virus ecodes a protein kinase associated with a phosphoprotein. Cell 15:561.

Lipsich, LA, Cutt J, Brugge JS (1982). Association of the transforming proteins of Rous, Fujinami and Y73 avian sarcoma viruses with the same two cellular proteins. Mol Cell Biol, in press.

McGrath JP, Levinson AD (1982). Bacterial expression of an enzymatically active protein encoded by RSV src gene. Nature 295:423-425.

Oppermann H, Levinson W, Bishop JM (1981). A cellular protein that associates with a transforming protein of Rous sarcoma virus is also a heat-shock protein. Proc Natl Acad Sci USA 78:1067.

Oppermann H, Levinson AD, Levintow L, Varmus HE, Bishop JM, Kawai S (1981). Two cellular proteins that immunoprecipitate with the transforming protein of Rous sarcoma virus. Virology 113:736.

Purchio AF, Erikson E, Brugge JS, Erikson RL (1978). Identification of a polypeptide encoded by the avian sarcoma virus src gene. Proc Natl Acad Sci USA 75:1567.

Purchio AF, Jonanovich S, Erikson RL (1980). Sites of synthesis of viral proteins in avian sarcoma virus-infected chicken cells. J Virol 35:629.

Sefton BM, Hunter T, Beemon K, Eckhart W (1980). Evidence that the phosphorylation of tyrosine is essential for cellular transformation by Rous sarcoma virus. Cell 20:807.

Weber MJ, Friis RR (1979) Dissociation of transformation parameters using temperature-conditional mutants of Rous sarcoma virus. Cell 16:25.

Oncogenes and Retroviruses: Evaluation of Basic Findings
and Clinical Potential, pages 149–157
© 1983 Alan R. Liss, Inc., 150 Fifth Avenue, New York, NY 10011

STUDIES ON THE 38 000 D PUTATIVE TARGET PROTEIN OF THE ROUS
SARCOMA VIRUS SRC GENE PRODUCT: ASSOCIATION WITH A CYTOSO-
LIC MALIC DEHYDROGENASE ISOENZYME

Helga Rübsamen[1], Peter Centner[1], Erich Eigenbrodt[2]
and Robert R. Friis[3]
[1]Paul-Ehrlich-Institut, D-6000 Frankfurt/M. 70
[2]Institut für Biochemie und Endokrinologie
 D-6300 Giessen
[3]Institut für Virologie, FB Humanmedizin,
 D-6300 Giessen, FRG

Rous sarcoma virus is an acutely-transforming avian retrovirus, which carries a host-derived oncogene within the
viral genome. The product of this gene, pp60^{src}, is a phosphoprotein of 60,000 d (Brugge and Erikson, 1977), which exhibits an unusual protein kinase activity (Collett and Erikson, 1978), phosphorylating tyrosine (Hunter and Sefton,
1980).

In an effort to study the role of host protein phosphorylation in oncogenic transformation, alterations in the
pattern of protein phosphorylation during transformation
were examined. The most prominent change in phosphorylation
upon transformation was found in a protein of 34,000 - 36,000
d (Radke and Martin, 1979; Erikson and Erikson, 1980).
Although remaining constant in amount, this protein showed
a 10 - 20 fold increase in phosphorylation, mainly in tyrosine. This change occured within one hour after the onset of
transformation. The protein appeared to be abundant, unglyco-
sylated, cytosolic and conserved in evolution. It was found
to have a pI-value of about 7.5.

The transformed state induced by Rous sarcoma virus is
characterized by increased lactic acid production (Carroll
et al., 1978). It has been argued that such a change may be
due to the increased uptake of glucose (Rambeck et al., 1975)
or to the enhanced utilization of glutamate by the cells
(Fodge and Rubin, 1975). Another possibility, not tested so
far with Rous sarcoma virus transformed cells, but which has
been described for human fibroblasts in culture, is that
the malate-aspartate shuttle transporting cytosolic reducing

equivalents into the mitochondria is diminished in rapidly
proliferating cells (Mc Keehan, 1982; Mc Keehan and Mc Keehan, 1982; Nakano et al.,1982). In view of such indications
for an influence of transformation on intermediary metabolism, we decided to examine some prominent metabolic enzymes
as possible candidates for the 34,000 - 36,000 d putative
target of pp60^{src}.

Upon   performing a purification of the 34,000 -
36,000 d protein according to the procedure of Erikson and
Erikson (1980), we isolated a protein which in our hands
exhibited an apparent molecular weight of 38,000 d (38K).
The identity of this protein with the putative target of
pp60^{src} was demonstrated by its rapid phosphorylation in
temperature-sensitive transformation-defective mutant-in-
fected cells after shift to the permissive temperature for
transformation. The phosphorylation was found in serine and
tyrosine, the protein had a pI of 7.5, and was specifically
immunoprecipitated by antiserum against the putative target
protein (Erikson et al., 1981) generously made available to
us by Dr. R. Erikson. A cytosolic malic dehydrogenase (MDH)
activity was found to be associated with this protein (Rübsamen et al., 1982).

In order to further substantiate this observation,
that the 38K protein is associated with a cytosolic MDH, we
decided to investigate if all cytosolic MDH activity is
associated with 38K. Previous experiments had shown (Rübsamen et al., 1982) that a substantial amount of an alkaline
pI MDH was extracted using the lysis conditions described
by Erikson and Erikson (1980). An effort was, therefore,
made to eliminate the alkaline pI MDH at as early a stage
of purification as possible. Gentle lysis procedures (table
1: II, III), which avoid the rupture of mitochondria were
found unsatisfactory because of their low yield in cytosolic MDH. Furthermore, very little 38K protein could be extracted under these conditions, suggesting an association
of 38K with particulate structures.

Since, accoding to the data in table 1, the extraction
of 38K and MDH was dependent on mild detergent treatment,
further experiments were directed to removing the pI 9.3
enzyme after extraction. When extracts were subjected to
isoelectric focussing under non-denaturing conditions after
being passed through DEAE-Sephacel, a broad distribution of
38K (pI 5.5 to 7.8) and an inefficient separation from the

pI 9.3 MDH as demonstrated by a second cycle of focussing, were observed (data not shown).

Table 1:   Yield of MDH activities and 38K protein using different extraction protocols

lysis conditions [a]	MDH [b] total (mU/ml)	MDH [c] pI 9.3 (mU/ml)	MDH [c] pI 5.5-7.8 (mU/ml)	38K [d] (%)
I 10 mM Tris, 0.05%NP40, pH 7.2 (Erikson and Erikson, 1980)	800	600	200	100
II 0.25 M sucrose, 10 mM Tris, 1 mM Mg^{2+} pH 7.2, Dounce homogenization	60	0	60	10
III same buffer as in II, N2-pressure 120 bar, 30 min	80	0	80	12

a) All lysis procedures were followed by centrifugation at 100,000x$\underline{g}$ for 30 min; 38K and MDH were assayed in the supernatant.

b) Determined by measuring the conversion of malate to oxalacetate (Rübsamen et al., 1982) to exclude contribution to the activity from lactate dehydrogenase in the reaction oxalacetate→malate.

c) Determined after isoelectric focussing of lysate under non-denaturing conditions.

d) Estimated by immunoprecipitation with antiserum (Erikson et al., 1981). The amount of 38K using condition I was defined as 100 %.

The quantitative removal of the alkaline MDH was finally achieved by chromatography on 5'-AMP-Sepharose (Fig.1)
(Rotmans, 1978).

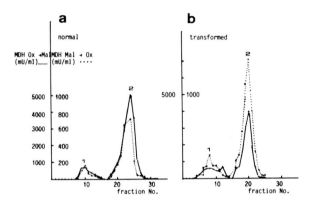

Fig. 1. Chromatography of cell lysates on 5'-AMP-Sepharose.
Chicken embryo cells infected with the NY68 temperature-
sensitive mutant of Rous sarcoma virus (Kawai and Hanafusa,
1971) and grown at 42° C (a) or shifted for 4 h to the permissive temperature for transformation (35° C, b) were lysed
in 20 mM potassium phosphate, 1 mM EDTA, 1 mM ß-mercapto-
ethanol, 1 mM NaF and 0.05 % Triton X-100 and centrifuged
at 100,000xg for 30 min. 50 ml of each lysate (0.8 mg pro-
tein/ml) were passed through a column filled with DEAE-Sephacel (1.5 x 4 cm) and then loaded onto a 1 x 7 cm column
containing 5'-AMP-Sepharose (Deutsche Pharmacia). The column
was developed with a linear gradient of NaCl. Peak I: flow-
through together with gradient up to 30 mM NaCl; Peak 2,
180 mM NaCl. MDH activity is shown.

The MDH activities eluting from 5'-AMP-Sepharose were
further characterized by isoelectric focussing under non-
denaturing conditions. The early fractions (peak I) contained MDH (pI 5.5 to 7.8) and 90 % of the 38K protein. In contrast, the enzyme eluting at 180 mM salt focussed in a sharp
peak at pI 9.3, and only traces of 38K were found associated
(data not shown). The distribution of MDH activity and 38K
protein in additional purification steps and the analysis of
some peak fractions on SDS polyacrylamide gels is shown in
Figs. 2 and 3.

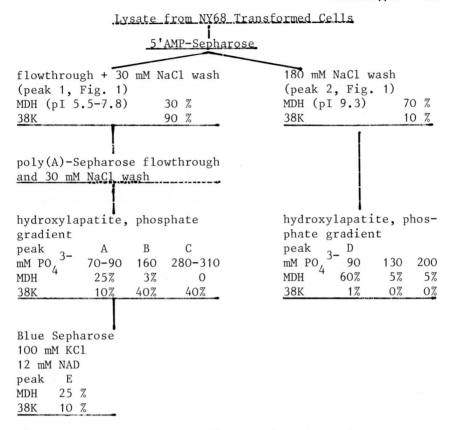

Fig. 2. Chromatography of 38K protein and MDH isoenzymes:
flow-diagram.
The MDH activities and the amount of 38K protein
are given as % of the lysate total. Blue Sepharose
chromatography was performed at pH 7.5, under
which conditions 38K and MDH are retained, in
contrast to previous experience at pH 8.6
(Rübsamen et al., 1982).

After passage through poly(A)-Sepharose and removal of
lactic dehydrogenase and glyceraldehyde-3-phosphate dehydrogenase (Rübsamen et al., 1982), the 38K protein chromato-
graphed in three peaks over hydroxylapatite. Most of the pI
5.5 - 7.8 MDH activity, and approximately 10 % of the total
38K protein eluted at low phosphate concentrations (peak A),
while the remaining 38K, eluted in peaks B and C was
associated with little MDH activity. Upon further purification

of peak A using chromatography on Blue Sepharose, virtually
pure 38K was eluted with 12 mM NAD in 100 mM KCl, coincident
with quantitative recovery of MDH activity (peak E).

Fig. 3 compares some peak fractions (as designated in
Fig. 2) for their behaviour on SDS polyacrylamide gel electrophoresis with commercially available pigeon breast muscle
MDH (Sigma). Fig. 3 (track C) shows the 38K eluting at
310 mM PO_4^{3-} from hydroxyapatite, corresponding to the peak
prepared by Erikson and Erikson, (1980). In track E the identical migration of enzymatically (MDH) active material eluting early from hydroxyapatite, and further purified over
Blue Sepharose (peak E) is demonstrated. In contrast, the pI
9.3 MDH prepared on 5'AMP-Sepharose chromatography (Fig. 3,
track D) exhibits a lower apparent molecular weight, essentially identical to that of the pigeon breast muscle MDH.
Like the pI 9.3 MDH enzyme purified from fibroblasts described in this communications, the MDH from pigeon breast
muscle exhibited a pI of 9.3 upon isoelectric focussing
(data not shown).

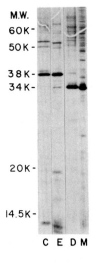

Fig. 3. SDS-polyacrylamide
gel electrophoresis of column
fractions and commercial MDH.
The samples were analyzed on
12 % SDS-polyacrylamide gels,
proteins were visualized by
staining with silver (Oakley
et al., 1980).
C, D, E: 15 µl of peak fractions as indicated in
Fig. 2.
M: MDH from pigeon breast
muscle (Sigma) 30 ng

The finding of two different isoenzymes of MDH in chick embryo cells is in agreement with results from many other laboratories. In contrast to bacteria, all eucaryotes appear to posess at least two isoenzymatic forms of MDH, the mitochondrial enzyme in most cases with alkaline pI value and the cytosolic enzyme with neutral or acidic pI (Banaszak and Bradshaw, 1975). Comparison of the amino acid composi‐tions of cytosolic and mitochondrial enzymes from yeast has shown that the enzymes differ to an extent which suggests that they are coded for by different, most likely evolutionarily divergent, genes (Hägele et al., 1978).

The results shown above indicate that mild detergent extraction of chicken embryo fibroblasts also yielded two different isoenzymes of MDH, the alkaline, presumably mitochondrial enzyme accounting for 70 - 80 % of the activity in the extract. All of the remaining activity was associated with a 38K phosphoprotein. This 38K protein can clearly be separated from two 38K forms with little MDH activity. It is so far unclear what the relation between the 38K protein associated with MDH activity, and the 38K protein exhibiting little activity, may be. Studies on their degree of relatedness and their sites of phosphorylation in normal and transformed cells are now in progress.

Our observation that the 38K phosphoprotein was associated with a cytosolic MDH activity (Rübsamen et al., 1982) has been questioned on the grounds that commercially available MDH does not co-migrate on polyacrylamide gel electrophoresis with the putative target of pp60^{src}. We show here that the commercial pigeon breast muscle MDH does co-migrate with the pI 9.3 MDH from chicken embryo cells;furthermore, that the pigeon breast muscle enzyme itself exhibits a pI of 9.3. The cytosolic isoenzyme, pI 5.5 - 7.8 from chicken embryo cells, however, which owing to its subunit molecular weight of 38,000 d and temperature-sensitive phosphorylation in cells infected by Rous sarcoma virus mutants has been suggested as a target for the pp60^{src}, is readily distinguishable.

ACKNOWLEDGEMENTS. We would like to thank Drs. Brede, Kurth, and Schoner for support and helpful discussions, and Dr. H. Bauer for critically reading the manuscript.
The financial support of these investigations by the Deutsche Forschungsgemeinschaft (Ru 242: H.R.; SFB 47: R.R.

F.; and Scho 139/15: E. E.) is gratefully acknowledged.

Banaszak LJ, Bradshaw RA (1975). Dehydrogenase. In Boyer PD (ed): The Enzymes. Vol. 11, New York: Academic Press, p 369.

Brugge JS, Erikson RL (1977). Identification of a transformation-specific antigen induced by an avian sarcoma virus. Nature 269:346.

Carroll RC, Ash JF, Vogt PK, Singer SJ (1978). Reversion of transformed glycolysis to normal by inhibition of protein synthesis in rat kidney cells infected with temperature-sensitive mutant of Rous sarcoma virus. Proc. Natl. Acad. Sci. USA 75:5015.

Collett MS, Erikson RL (1978). Protein kinase activity associated with the avian sarcoma virus src gene product. Proc. Natl. Acad. Sci. USA 75:2021.

Erikson, E, Erikson RL (1980). Identification of a cellular substrate phosphorylated by the avian sarcoma virus src gene product. Cell 21:829.

Erikson E, Cook G, Miller J, Erikson RL (1981). The same normal cell protein is phosphorylated after transformation by avian sarcoma viruses with unrelated transforming genes. Mol. Cell. Biol. 1:43.

Fodge DW, Rubin H (1975). Stimulation of lactic production in chick embryo fibroblasts by serum and high pH in the absence of external glucose. J. Cell. Physiol. 86:453.

Hägele E, Neeff J, Mecke D (1978). The malate dehydrogenase isoenzymes of saccharomyces cerevisiae: Purification, characterization and studies on their regulation. Eur. J. Biochem. 83:67.

Hunter T, Sefton BM (1980). The transforming gene product of Rous sarcoma viruses phosphorylates tyrosine. Proc. Natl. Acad. Sci. USA 77:1311.

Kawai S, Hanafusa H (1971). The effects of the reciprocal changes in temperature on the transformed state of cells infected with a Rous sarcoma virus mutant. Virology 46: 470.

Mc Keehan WL (1982). Glycolysis, glutaminolysis and cell proliferation. In Cell Biology. International Reports, Vol. 6 (Academic Press, London); p.635.

Mc Keehan WL, Mc Keehan KA (1982): Changes in NAD(P)-dependent malic enzyme and malate dehydrogenase activities during fibroblast proliferation. J. Cell. Physiol. 110: 142.

Nakano ET, Ciampi NA, Young DV (1982): The identification of a serum viability factor for SV3T3 cells as biotin and its possible relationship to the maintenance of Krebs cycle activity. Arch. Biochem. Biophys. 215:556.

Oakley BR, Kirsch DR, Morris NR (1980). A simplified ultra-sensitive silver stain for detecting proteins in poly-acrylamide gels. Anal. Biochem. 105:361.

Radke K, Martin GS (1979). Transformation by Rous sarcoma virus: Effects of src gene expression on the synthesis and phosphorylation of cellular polypeptides. Proc. Natl. Acad. Sci. USA 76:5212.

Rambeck WA, Bissell MJ, Bassham JA (1975). Metabolism in normal and virus-transformed chick embryo fibroblasts as observed with glucose labeled with ^{14}C and tritium and with tritium-labeled water. Hoppe Seyler's Z. Physiol. Chem. 356:203.

Rotmans JP (1978). Schistosoma mansoni: Purification and characterization of malate dehydrogenases. Exp. Parasitology 46:31.

Rübsamen H, Saltenberger K, Friis RR, Eigenbrodt E (1982). Cytosolic malic dehydrogenase activity is associated with a putative substrate for the transforming gene product of Rous sarcoma virus. Proc. Natl. Acad. Sci. USA 79:228.

Oncogenes and Retroviruses: Evaluation of Basic Findings
and Clinical Potential, pages 159–169
© 1983 Alan R. Liss, Inc., 150 Fifth Avenue, New York, NY 10011

THE REGULATION OF A CELLULAR PROTEIN, P53, IN NORMAL AND TRANSFORMED CELLS

Arnold J. Levine, Nancy Reich and Rees Thomas

State University of New York at Stony Brook
Department of Microbiology-School of Medicine
Stony Brook, New York 11794

Cells transformed by a wide variety of agents contain elevated levels of a 53,000 molecular weight cellular phosphoprotein, termed p53 (DeLeo et al., 1979; Lane and Crawford, 1979; Linzer and Levine, 1979). Antibodies to this protein, which have been employed to identify and quantitate it, were first detected in animals bearing simian virus 40 (SV40) induced tumors (Lane and Crawford, 1979; Linzer and Levine, 1979) or in mice hyperimmunized with syngeneic cells transformed with a chemical carcinogen (DeLeo et al., 1979). There are a number of reasons why the cellular encoded p53 protein appears to be interesting in understanding the mechanisms of cellular transformation. First, 10–100 fold higher levels of p53 have been detected in many transformed cells when compared to nontransformed cells. Such diverse transforming activities, as DNA tumor viruses (Linzer, Maltzman and Levine, 1979), RNA tumor viruses (DeLeo et al., 1979; Rotter, Boss and Baltimore, 1981), chemical carcinogens or physical agents such as irradiation (DeLeo et al., 1979) genetic predisposition giving rise to teratocarcinomas (Linzer and Levine, 1979) or spontaneous transformation events (3T12) (Maltzman, Oren and Levine, 1981), all can result in tumors or transformed cell lines expressing enhanced levels of the p53 antigen. Thus, the expression of this protein in high quantities is independent of the original transforming agents. Second, a similar p53 protein has been detected in mouse, rat, hamster, monkey and human cells (Linzer and Levine, 1979; Smith, Smith and Paucha, 1979; Simmons et al., 1980; Gurney et al., 1980; Crawford et al., 1981). Some monoclonal antibodies to the p53 protein from mice cross react with homologous p53 proteins in most or all of these species (Gurney et

al. 1980; Harlow et al., 1981) while other monoclonal antibodies are specific for primate p53 protein (Thomas, Sullivan
and Levine, unpublished results) or the murine p53 antigen
(Harlow et al., 1981). These results indicate the p53 molecules from different species share some common determinants
as well as contain species specific antigenic determinants.
Consistent with this is the observation that the p53 proteins
from human, monkey, mouse and rat share some, but not all,
methionine containing tryptic peptides in common (Simmons
et al., 1980). The p53 antigens isolated from different
transformed mouse cell lines appear to be similar or identical by tryptic peptide mapping, independent of the transforming agent (Maltzman et al., 1981). Thus, the p53 protein has been conserved over evolutionary time scales, perhaps indicating an essential function in cell growth or
development. Thirdly, in SV40 (Lane and Crawford, 1979;
Linzer and Levine, 1979) and adenovirus (Sarnow et al., 1982)
transformed mouse cell lines, the p53 antigen is physically
associated or found in a multimeric complex with the viral
encoded tumor antigens, known to be required for the transformation process. This association of a cellular protein
with the transforming viral gene products (tumor antigens)
suggests an involvement of p53 in the process of transformation.

   Given these indications that p53 may play a role in
transformation, several interesting questions, concerning
the properties of this protein, may now be asked. How are
the levels of p53 regulated in nontransformed and transformed cells? What is the function of p53 in normal cells
and how is this altered in transformed cells? These questions have been studied employing several diverse systems
such as SV40 and adenovirus transformed cells, embryonal
carcinoma cells differentiating into nontransformed endo-
derm-like cells, and nontransformed 3T3 cells synchronized
to study events in the cell cycle. This paper will review
these studies and attempt to bring together these observations into a conceptual framework for understanding the role
of p53 in the normal and transformed cell.

SIMIAN VIRUS 40

   In SV40 transformed cells, the SV40 large T-antigen is
physically complexed with the cellular p53 protein (Lane

and Crawford, 1979; Levine and Linzer, 1979). Monoclonal antibodies specific for the SV40 large T-antigen (Gurney et al., 1980) immunoprecipitate the SV40 T-antigen and coimmuno-precipitate the associated p53 protein (Linzer and Levine, 1979). Similarly, monoclonal antibodies specific for the murine p53 antigen (Jay et al., 1981) immunoprecipitate p53 and coimmunoprecipitate the associated viral T-antigen (Maltzman et al., 1981). Temperature sensitive mutants (SV40tsA mutants) in the structural gene for the viral large T-antigen, regulate the levels of cellular p53 in a tempera-ture dependent fashion in virus infected or transformed cells (Linzer et al., 1979). Thus, the viral T-antigen directly or indirectly controls the levels of cellular p53 in cells. The SV40 large T-antigen also regulates the maintenance of the transformed state (Brockman, 1978) and so p53 levels and the transformed phenotype of a cell line are both affected by the same viral protein. In nontransformed cells, the p53 pro-tein is synthesized but is rapidly degraded so that this pro-tein has a half life of only 20 to 30 minutes in 3T3 cells. This results in low levels of p53 being detected in nontrans-formed cells (Oren et al., 1981). In SV40 transformed cells, the half life of the p53 protein is greater than 22 hours, leading to the accumulation and high levels of p53 in these cells (Oren et al., 1981). These differences in post-trans-lational control of p53 can explain the higher levels of p53 in SV40 transformed cells compared with nontransformed cells. The levels of translatable p53 mRNA in 3T3 cells or SV40 transformed 3T3 cells are about equal, indicating that the rate of synthesis of p53 in these two cells may be similar (Oren et al., 1981). Thus it appears that the levels of p53, in SV40 transformed 3T3 cells, can be regulated at the post-translational, or protein stability level. The enhanced stability of p53 in SV40 transformed cells could result from the binding of T-antigen to p53, reducing p53 turnover (Oren et al., 1981) or from T-antigen induced post-translational modifications of p53, providing it greater stability (Maltz-man et al., 1981).

The prolonged half life or stability of p53 in cells transformed by agents other than SV40 may also explain, at least in part, the higher levels of p53 found in transformed cells. While 3T3 cells regulate p53 with a half life of 20-30 minutes, F9 embryonal carcinoma cells and methylcholan-threne transformed 3T3 cells (Meth A) contain p53 proteins with half lives of 3 hours and 5 hours respectively (Reich and Levine, unpublished results). Other means of regulating

p53 are also possible (Oren, Reich and Levine, 1981) and may
play a combined role in determining the final levels of p53
detected in these cells.

ADENOVIRUSES

     In adenovirus transformed mouse, rat or hamster cells,
the viral E1b-58K tumor antigen is physically complexed with
the cellular p53 protein (Sarnow et al., 1982). Monoclonal
antibodies directed against p53 coimmunoprecipitate the
viral E1b-58K protein. Similarly, monoclonal antibodies
directed against the E1b-58K tumor antigen coimmunoprecipitate the cellular p53 protein (Sarnow, Sullivan and Levine,
1982). The adenovirus DNA sequences contained in the early
region E1a and E1b genes are sufficient for transformation
of cells in culture (Graham et al., 1974). Point mutations
and deletions in the E1b genes prevent the virus from transforming rat cell in culture (Graham et al., 1978; Jones and
Shenk, 1979). Thus the adenovirus E1b-58K tumor antigen
may play a role in viral transformation and is detected in
a physical association with cellular p53 protein.

     The E1b-58K-p53 complex and the SV40 large T-p53 complex
share a number of properties in common. Both complexes are
heterogeneous in size or mass and are composed of multimeric
combinations of the viral and cellular proteins (McCormick
and Harlow, 1980; Sarnow et al., 1982). In both the adenovirus and SV40 T-antigen-p53 complexes, most or all of the
detectable p53 is found in the high molecular weight complex with little or no free p53 found in the cell extract
(Sarnow et al., 1982). In addition, the adenovirus E1b-58K
protein and the SV40 large T-antigen share several functions
in common. Both antigens are required for transformation
of cells with a complete transformed phenotype (Tegtmeyer,
1975; Jones and Shenk, 1979). The SV40 large T-antigen
(Tegtmeyer, 1972) and the adenovirus E1b-58K protein are
both involved in the replication of viral DNA (Ross et al.,
1980) and both viral proteins can modulate the levels of
several early viral gene products during productive infection (Alwine, Reed and Stark, 1977; Ross et al., 1980).
Thus, the functions of these viral proteins in viral DNA
replication and gene regulation may be acted upon by p53
resulting in some facets of the transformed state. It remains possible, but not proven, that the association of the

adenovirus Elb-58K antigen with p53, could stabilize this
protein, resulting in an increased half life and enhanced
levels in transformed cells.

EMBRYONAL CARCINOMA CELLS

     Embryonal carcinoma cells contain higher levels of p53
than a variety of nontransformed cell lines (Linzer and Levine, 1979). F9 embryonal carcinoma cells are fully transformed and tumorigenic in syngeneic mice. When exposed to
retinoic acid and dibutyrl cyclic AMP these cells differentiate in culture into endoderm which no longer forms tumors
in animals and does not express any transformed properties
(Strickland and Mahdavi, 1978; Strickland, Smith and Marotli,
1980). After differentiation of F9 embryonal carcinoma cells
into endoderm, the levels of p53 in these cells falls 5-10
fold (Oren et al., 1982). The half life of p53 protein in
both F9 cells and endoderm cells remains the same,however,
about 3-3.5 hours. Thus a change in protein stability cannot account for the decline in the levels of p53 upon differentiation and reversion of the transformed state (Oren et
al., 1982). Instead the levels of p53 translatable mRNA's
detected in endoderm cells was about 6-10 fold lower than
in equivalent RNA preparations (same concentration of total
RNA) from F9 embryonal carcinoma cells (Oren et al., 1982).
In this system it appears that p53 is regulated by the levels of mRNA present in the cells. Whether this is due to
a transcriptional regulation or an alteration in the stability of p53 mRNA in these cells remains to be determined.

P53 REGULATION DURING THE CELL CYCLE

     Several lines of evidence indicate that p53 levels in
normal cells may be altered by cell division or active cell
growth. Higher levels of p53 were detected in mitogen
stimulated lymphocytes (Milner and McCormick, 1980; Milner
and Milner, 1981). Higher than expected levels of p53 were
found in normal thymocytes (Jay et al., 1980; Rotter et al.,
1981) an organ involved in active cell division in young
animals. Finally, p53 synthesis was readily detected in
explants of early embryos at specific stages of growth or
development (Mora, Chandrasekaran and MacFarland, 1980).
These observations have led to a study of the synthesis
of p53 during the cell cycle (Reich and Levine, unpublished

results).

In 3T3 cells synchronized by serum deprivation, the addition of fresh serum induces the cells to enter into the S-phase (by 12-15 hours after addition of serum) and cell division (by 20 hours). In these cells p53 levels increase 4-6 fold both before the start of S-period and into the DNA synthetic period. The p53 levels then decline along with the declining rate of DNA synthesis as cells move into the G-2 period (Reich and Levine, unpublished observations). When cellular DNA synthesis is blocked by an inhibitor such as hydroxyurea, the p53 levels increase with time after serum stimulation, indicating that DNA synthesis itself, is not responsible for this rise in p53 production. The half lives of the p53 protein synthesized in early G-1 or the S-phase are both about 20 minutes so that the increased p53 levels observed in late G-1 and S are not due to an enhanced stability of this protein. It appears likely then that the rate of synthesis of p53 molecules increases in late G-1 and S phase, presumably reflecting its function at this time. Smaller increases in the levels of p53 can also be observed shortly after serum is added to the 3T3 cultures (Reich and Levine, unpublished results). These studies indicate that p53 may play a role in regulating events in the cell cycle which can then be altered in the transformed cell by longer p53 half lives and the association of p53 with viral tumor antigens.

STEADY STATE LEVELS OF P53 IN HUMAN CELL LINES

The studies reviewed here suggest that the p53 protein may play a central role in the transformation process independent of the transforming agent. If this presumption is correct, then p53 levels should be a good measure of transformation or tumorigenesis in human malignancies. Indeed, Crawford et al., (1981) have detected elevated levels of p53 in a wide variety of human carcinomas, lymphomas and leukemias in cell culture. Because the amount of p53 in a cell appears to be regulated at both mRNA and post-translational levels, depending upon the system under study, the metabolic labeling of p53 proteins in cell culture for a defined time period may not reflect the steady state levels of this protein in cells. Thus, comparing p53 levels in cells with different half lives of p53 could lead to an under or over estimate of p53 levels depending upon the

length of time chosen for the labeling of p53 with radio-
active precursor molecules. For this reason, the radioim-
munometric assay developed by Lane, Gannon and Winchester
(1982) was modified and employed to measure the steady state
levels of p53 in human cells derived from tumors or trans
formed in culture. Primate specific or reactive monoclonal
antibodies were employed (Thomas, Sullivan and Levine, unpublished results and Harlow et al., 1981) in the radioim-
munometric assay. The steady state levels of p53 were determined in SV80 cells, primary human cells transformed by
SV40 (Todaro, Green and Swift, 1966), Raji cells, an EBV
positive Burkitt lymphoma cell line (Pulvertaft, 1964), a
human melanoma cell line (from D. Rifkin), Tera I, a human
testicular teratocarcinoma (Fough and Trempe, 1975), the
IB-4 cell line, normal human chord lymphocytes transformed
by EBV (King et al., 1980) and normal WI38 primary human
fibroblasts in culture (Hayflick and Moorhead, 1961). Purified p53 from SV80 cells was employed to standardize the
protein levels of p53 detected by this assay (Thomas and
Levine, unpublished results). Table 1 presents the results
determining the steady state levels of p53 in these tumor
derived and transformed cell lines.

Table 1

P53 Levels in Human Cell Lines

Cell lines	P53 ugms/gram cell protein
SV80	450
Raji	11
Melanoma	10
Tera 1	3.3
IB4	1.6
WI38	<0.2

The SV80 cells contained greater than 2000 fold more p53
than normal cells. The other tumor derived and transformed
cell lines contained between greater than 8-55 fold more p53
than WI38 cells. It appears likely, based upon the studies
reviewed here, that SV40 transformed cells contain very high
levels of p53 because the SV40 T-antigen stabilizes this
protein and provides a very long half life (>22 hours) while
embryonal carcinoma cells (half life 3-3.5 hrs) lie between
this extreme and nontransformed cells (3T3, 20-30 minutes).

It is of some interest that a Burkitt lymphoma line carrying EBV DNA (Raji) contained about 10 fold more p53 than a
normal chord lymphocyte transformed in vitro by EBV (IB4).
While this sample is too small to make any firm conclusions
this result is of some interest in possibly distinguishing
between tumorigenesis and transformation in vitro. It is
clear from these studies, that the steady state levels of
human p53, like those in the mouse system, are correlated
with transformation and tumorigenesis.

CONCLUSIONS

   In nontransformed 3T3 cells p53 levels appear to be regulated by or with the cell cycle. The amount of p53 detected increases prior to S-phase and reaches a maximum in
S-phase. In SV40 and adenovirus transformed cells the viral
tumor antigens can be found physically associated with p53
(Lane and Crawford, 1979; Linzer and Levine, 1979; Sarnow et
al., 1982). The SV40 large T-antigen can stimulate cells to
enter the S-period when microinjected into these cells
(Tjian, Fey and Grossman, 1978). As a reasonable hypothesis,
then, we would suggest that p53 in nontransformed cells plays
a role in regulating the entry of cells into S-phase. During
this process p53 is required in small amounts and is regulated by a rapid turnover of the protein (20-30 minute half
life) (Oren et al., 1981). In SV40 transformed cells T-antigen binds to and stabilizes p53 resulting in increased
levels of this protein and forcing the cells into S-phase
under inappropriate conditions. This gives rise to the
transformed phenotype where cells replicate with an altered
growth control. In embryonal carcinoma cells (half life of
p53 is 3-3.5 hrs) or methylcholanthrene transformed cells
(half life of p53 is 5 hrs) higher levels of p53 also could
give rise to altered growth characteristic termed the transformed phenotype. P53 levels can also be regulated at the
transcriptional or mRNA stability level as seen in the F9
embryonal carcinoma system (Oren et al., 1982). A protein,
p53, that normally turns over rapidly appears to be a good
candidate for a regulatory element in the cell cycle.
Transforming agents alter the regulation of the cell cycle,
possibly at one or more places. The increased levels of
p53 detected in tumorigenic and transformed cells could in
some cases be causative and in other situations reflect this
altered growth control. The net result is the higher levels
of p53 detected in the human transformed or tumorigenic cell

lines (table 1) might then reflect different primary events leading to altered cell growth and resulting in higher p53 levels than detected in normal WI38 cells. Whatever the role of p53 in regulating cell replication, it appears that the function of this protein in the cell cycle could be important to our understanding of normal and abnormal cellular processes.

REFERENCES

Alwine JC, Reed SI, Stark GR (1977). Characterization of the autoregulation of simian virus 40 gene A. J Virol 24:22-29.

Brockman WW (1978). Transformation of balb/c 3T3 cells by tsA mutants of SV40 temperature sensitivity of the transformed phenotype and retransformation of wild type virus. J Virol 25:860-868.

Crawford, LV, Pim DC, Gurney EG, Goodfellow P, Taylor-Papadimitriou J (1981). Detection of a common feature in several human tumor cell lines: a 53,000 dalton protein. Proc Natl Acad Sci (USA) 78:41-45.

DeLeo AB, Jay G, Appella E, Dubois GC, Law LW, Old LJ (1979). Detection of a transformation related antigen in chemically induced sarcomas and other transformed cells of the mouse. Proc Natl Acad Sci (USA) 76:2420-2424.

Fough J, Trempe G (1975). "Human Tumor Cells In Vitro" New York: Plenum

Graham FL, Abrahams PJ, Mulder C, Heyneker HL, Warnaar SO, DeVries KAJ, Fiers W, van der Eb AJ (1974). Studies on in vitro transformation by DNA and DNA fragments of human adenoviruses and simian virus 40. Cold Spr Harbor Symp Quant Biol 39:637-650.

Graham FL, Harrison T, Williams J (1978). Defective Transforming capacity of adenovirus type 5 host range mutants. Virol 86:10-12.

Gurney EG, Harrison RO, Fenno J (1980) Monoclonal antibodies against simian virus 40 T-antigens: evidence for distinct subclasses of large T-antigen and similarities among nonviral T-antigen. J Virol 34:752-763.

Harlow E, Crawford LV, Pim DC, Williamson NM (1981). Monoclonal antibodies specific for simian virus 40 tumor antigens. J Virol 38:861-869

Jay G, Khoury G, DeLeo AB, Dippold WG, Old LJ (1981). p53 transformation-related protein:detection of an associated phosphotransferase activity. Proc Natl Acad Sci (USA) 78:2932-2936

Jones N, Shenk T (1979). Isolation of adenovirus type 5 host range deletion mutants defective for transformation in rat embryo cells. Cell 17:683-689.

King W, Thomas-Powell AL, Raab-Traub N, Hawke N, Kieff E (1980). Epstein Barr Virus RNA V viral RNA in a restringently infected growth transformed cell line. J Virol 36: 506-518.

Lane DP, Crawford LV (1979). T-antigen is bound to a host protein in SV40 transformed cells. Nature 278:261-263.

Lane DP, Gannon J, Winchester G (1982) The complex between p53 and SV40 T antigen. In Klein G (ed) "Advances In Viral Oncology 2", New York: Raven Press.

Linzer DIH, Levine AJ (1979). Characterization of a 54K dalton cellular SV40 tumor antigen present in SV40-transformed cells and uninfected embryonal carcinoma cells. Cell 17:43-52.

Linzer DIH, Maltzman W, Levine AJ (1979). The SV40 A gene product is required for the production of a 54,000 mw cellular tumor antigen. Virol 98:308-318.

Maltzman W, Oren M, Levine AJ (1981). The structural relationships between 54,000 molecular weight cellular tumor antigens detected in viral and nonviral transformed cells. Virol 112:145-156.

McCormick F, Harlow E (1980). Association of a murine 53,000 dalton phosphoprotein with simian virus 40 large T-antigen in transformed cells. J Virol 34: 213-224.

Milner J, McCormick F (1980). Lymphocyte stimulation: Concanvalin A induces the expression of a 53K protein. Cell Biol Int Rep 4:663-667.

Milner J, Milner S (1981). SV40 53K antigen: a possible role for 53K in normal cells. Virol 112:785-788.

Mora PT, Chandrasekaran K, McFarland VW (1980). An embryo protein induced by SV40 virus transformation of mouse cells. Nature 288:722-724.

Oren M, Maltzman W, Levine AJ (1981). Post-translational regulation of the 54K cellular tumor antigen in normal and transformed cells. Mol & Cell Biol 1:101-110.

Oren M, Reich N, Levine AJ (1982). The regulation of the cellular p53 tumor antigen in teratocarcinoma cells and their differentiated progeny. J Cell & Mol Bio 2:443-449.

Pulvertaft RJV (1964). Cytology of Burkitt's lymphoma. Lancet 1:238-240.

Ross SR, Levine AJ, Galos RS, Williams SJ, Shenk T (1980) Early viral proteins in HeLa cells infected with adenovirus type 5 host range mutants. Virol 103:475-492.

Rotter V, Boss MA, Baltimore D (1981). Increased concentration of an apparently identical cellular protein in cells transformed by either Abelson murine leukemia virus or other transforming agents. J Virol 38:336-346.

Sarnow P, Ho YS, Williams J, Levine AJ (1982). Adenovirus E1b-58Kd tumor antigen and SV40 large tumor antigen are physically associated with the same 54Kd cellular protein in transformed cells. Cell 28:387-394.

Sarnow P, Sullivan CA, Levine AJ (1982). A monoclonal antibody detecting the adenovirus type 5 E1b-58Kd tumor antigen: Characterization of the E1b-58Kd tumor antigen in adenovirus infected and transformed cells. Virol 120: 510-517.

Simmons DT, Martin MA, Mora PT, Chang C (1980). Relationship among Tau antigens isolated from various lines of simian virus 40 transformed cells. J Virol 34:650-657.

Smith AE, Smith R, Paucha E (1979). Characterization of different tumor antigens present in cells transformed by simian virus 40. Cell 18:335-346.

Strickland S, Mahdavi V (1978). The induction of differentiation in teratocarcinoma stem cells by retinoic acid. Cell 15:393-403.

Strickland S, Smith KE, Marotti KR (1980). Hormonal Induction of differentiation in teratocarcinoma stem cells: generation of parietal endoderm by retinoic acid and dibutyril cAMP. Cell 21:347-355.

Tegtmeyer P (1972). Simian virus 40 deoxyribonucleic acid synthesis: the viral replicon. J Virol 10:591-598.

Tegtmeyer P (1975). The function of simian virus 40 gene A in transforming infection. J Virol 15:613-618.

Tjian R, Fey G, Graessmann A (1978). Biological activity of purified simian virus 40 T-antigen proteins. Proc Natl Acad Sci(USA) 75:1279-1283.

Todaro G, Green H, Swift M (1966). Susceptibility of human diploid fibroblast strains to transformation by SV40 virus. Science 153:1252-1254.

ONC GENE AND HUMAN NEOPLASIA

**Oncogenes and Retroviruses: Evaluation of Basic Findings
and Clinical Potential, pages 173–183**
© 1983 Alan R. Liss, Inc., 150 Fifth Avenue, New York, NY 10011

STUDIES OF CLONED GENES FOR A SURFACE ANTIGEN CORRELATED
WITH HUMAN CHRONIC LYMPHOCYTIC LEUKEMIA

C.P. Stanners*, J.W. Chamberlain*, T. Lam and
G.B. Price[†]

The Ontario Cancer Institute
500 Sherbourne St.
Toronto, Ontario, Canada M4X 1K9

Present addresses: Dept. of Biochemistry* and
Cancer Centre[†], McGill University, 3655 Drummond
St., Montreal, P.Q., Canada H3G 1Y6.

We have recently reported the cloning of two genes,
HSAG-1 and HSAG-2, which are capable of determining a cell
surface antigen correlated with human chronic lymphocytic
leukemia (Stanners et al., 1981). The antigen can be
detected with a monoclonal antibody (37) which reacts with
5-30% of nucleated cells from peripheral blood or bone
marrow of patients with CLL and B-cell lymphomas; the
antibody does not react with normal human lymphocytes or
cells from patients with the various forms of acute leukemia
or a large number of cell lines, including some human
embryonic cell lines. The HSAG genes were isolated from a
gene library of a Chinese hamster-human CLL hybrid cell
(HCH-1), using their ability to transform L-strain mouse
cells to produce surface antigen and to cause morphological
transformation together with the presence of human-specific,
highly reiterated sequences (Gusella et al., 1980) as a
means of identification. Recent experiments point to a
rather surprising conclusion: these genes are part of a
large gene family, with dispersed nucleotide sequences,
variable flanking sequences, and copy numbers in the
thousands - properties which categorize it unequivocally as
middle repetitive DNA. This article contains some of the
early evidence in support of such a conclusion.

HSAG IS A MIDDLE REPETITIVE GENE FAMILY

Functional Gene Copy Number

     During the cloning of HSAG-1 and HSAG-2, it was found
that relatively strong antigen producers, such as HSAG-1,
were present in the gene library of HCH-1 at a frequency of
about one in every 10^4 clones which, for this library, gives
a copy number of about 100 per cell genome. Weaker antigen
producers, such as HSAG-2, were about 10 times more frequent,
giving a copy number of 1000 per cell genome (Stanners et
al., 1981). This result did not surprise us at first
because HCH-1 was a human CLL-Chinese hamster hybrid cell
selected for an extremely rounded cellular morphology, a
selection which could have resulted in amplification of
antigen determining genes, much as toxic drug selection can
result in amplification of genes for drug resistance (Alt
et. al, 1978).

Analysis of HSAG Family by Southern Gels of Genomic DNA

     A restriction map of HSAG-1, updated from our
previously published map (Stanners et al., 1981), is shown
in Fig. 1.

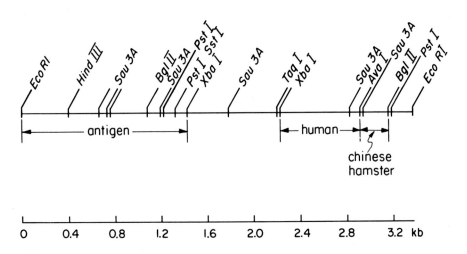

Fig. 1 Restriction map of HSAG-1.

The detailed structure of HSAG-1 including its nucleotide sequence, will be presented elsewhere. For the purpose of this article, only its salient features need be mentioned. The highly repetitive human-specific nucleotide sequence which was partially responsible for the isolation of HSAG-1 from the HCH-1 gene library is at the right hand end of the molecule, immediately adjacent to a Chinese hamster-specific highly repetitive sequence. We suggest that recombination between such sequences was responsible for the integration of HSAG-1 into the hybrid cell genome. The antigen-determining portion of HSAG-1 was determined by transformation of L cells with fragments isolated from electrophoretic gels, and was found to be in the left hand end of the molecule within the EcoRl and XbaI sites. Removal of the far left EcoRl to Hind III piece (417 bp) greatly reduced antigen production, while removal of the far right SstI to XbaI piece (120 bp) in addition, obliterated antigen production. No other portion of the molecule showed any ability to produce antigen. The nucleotide sequence of the 1440 bp EcoRl-XbaI fragment shows conventional transcriptional initiation and termination signals with methionine initiator codons, open reading frames and introns sufficient to code for the estimated 28,000 daltons of protein comprising the antigen (unpublished results). This, coupled with our demonstration of poly A+ transcripts complementary to the EcoRl-XbaI fragment associated with polysomes (unpublished results) makes it very likely that this fragment codes directly for the antigen. We assume this to be true, but direct proof must await cell-free translation of the antigen using the EcoRl-XbaI-homologous transcripts.

The EcoRl-XbaI fragment was labelled by nick translation and used as a hybridization probe to detect homologous sequences in EcoRl-digested genomic DNA separated by electrophoresis on agarose gels and transferred to nitrocellulose sheets. Under stringent conditions of hybridization we obtained a predominant band at 3.7 kb (larger than HSAG-1, which is 3.4 kb) (Fig. 2, left) in a smear extending from about 2 kb to 20 kb (Fig. 2, right). The band was estimated to represent a copy number of about 100 per genome and had the same basic restriction map as HSAG-1 (data not shown). These results were obtained with both the HCH-1 hybrid cell and its Chinese hamster parent, L-73 or LR-73. DNA from human CLL cells showed basically similar results, but with less prominent bands (Fig. 2).

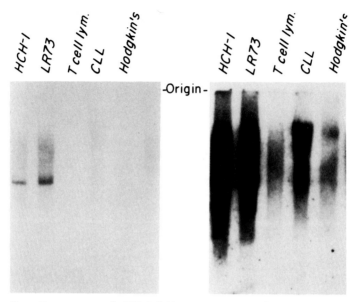

Fig. 2. Presence of HSAG-like sequences in various types
of genomic DNA. The latter were digested with EcoRl,
subject to electrophoresis on an agarose gel, and
transferred to nitrocellulose. HSAG-like sequences were
detected by hybridization with ^{32}P-labelled EcoRl-XbaI
fragment of HSAG-1. Left, short exposure to radioauto-
graphic film; right, long exposure.

We interpret these results to indicate the presence of a
family of reiterated HSAG-like sequences with approximately
the same configuration (the bands), in a much larger family
of reiterated sequences with less homology to HSAG-1 and
with varied configuration (the smear). HSAG-2, which is
9.5 kb in size (Stanners et al., 1981) has a region with
similar but non-identical restriction map to the EcoRl-XbaI
portion of HSAG-2. The similar regions of HSAG-1 and HSAG-2
require reduced stringency to hybridize (unpublished results).
HSAG-2 is therefore a more distant relative of HSAG-1 and
would presumably be represented in the smear. All of the
above places the HSAG family squarely in the domain of
classical middle repetitive sequences, as described for
example by Scheller et al. (1981) for sea urchin genomic
DNA.

Analysis of HSAG Family by Gene Libraries of Genomic DNA

Libraries of LR-73 (the Chinese hamster parent of HCH-1) and human CLL DNA were prepared by partial digestion of the DNA with EcoRl followed by ligation with λgtWES DNA digested with both EcoRl and SstI (SstI cuts the viral DNA insert in λgtWES twice, which reduces greatly the chance of reforming infectious DNA with viral inserts). The ligated DNA was packaged (Becker & Gold, 1975) and plated on appropriate bacteria to allow plaque formation, and the plaques transferred to nitrocellulose sheets. These were then denatured and hybridized with the ^{32}P-labelled EcoRl-XbaI fragment of HSAG-1 by the procedure of Benton & Davis (1978). Many of the plaques were labelled (Fig. 3).

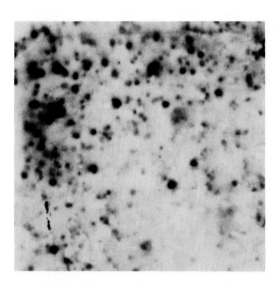

Fig. 3. Plaques of recombinant λ phage representative of LR-73 genomic DNA labelled by hybridization with the EcoRl-XbaI fragment of HSAG-1.

The quantitative results are shown in Table 1. Assuming that genomic DNA is represented randomly in the libraries, copy numbers of 10,000 to 30,000 of HSAG-like genes were calculated for the Chinese hamster cell genomes and 3,000 to 4,000 for the human CLL genome.

Table 1

FREQUENCY OF HSAG-1 R1-Xba-LIKE SEQUENCES
IN λ LIBRARIES

Library	% +ve Plaques	% +ve DNA	Copy No.
HCH-1	2.4%	0.6%	16,000
LR-73	7.1%	1.1%	28,000
CLL-1	0.94%	0.13%	3,400

Ten of the EcoRl-XbaI-positive plaques from the human CLL gene library were picked and amplified. DNA was purified from these clones, digested with EcoRl, subjected to electrophoresis on agarose gels and transferred to nitrocellulose sheets. The presence of HSAG-like DNA was assessed by hybridization with nick-translated EcoRl-XbaI fragment of HSAG-1. Typical results are shown in Figure 4. It can be seen that the size and number of inserted EcoRl fragments varied markedly from clone to clone; usually one of these fragments was labelled for each clone and the degree of labelling was markedly variable. These results are exactly what would be expected for a family of genes with dispersed base sequence and dispersed location in the genome.

The traditional definition of a reiterated gene family obtained from base sequence homology has the disadvantage that the size of the family depends arbitrarily on the conditions of hybridization. We were also aware that our results could be due to the presence of a sequence in one of the introns in the EcoRl-XbaI fragment which was reiterated to a much greater extent than the true antigen coding sequence. We therefore tested the human CLL clones for their ability to transform L TK$^-$ cells to produce antigen by the TK$^+$ HAT medium co-selection test described earlier (Stanners et al., 1981). Typical results are shown in Fig. 5. A summary of the results is shown in Table 2, including the degree of homology of the various inserts with the 0.79 kb XbaI-XbaI fragment of HSAG-1, which is immediately adjacent to the antigen-determining EcoRl-XbaI fragment (Figure 1).

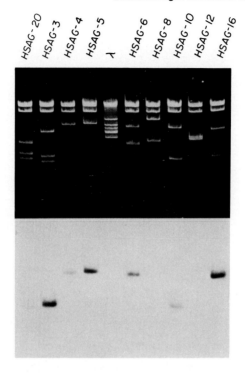

Fig. 4. Purified DNA from individual clones of human CLL
DNA in λ phage digested with EcoRl and subjected to
electrophoresis in 1% agarose gels.
Upper: ethidium bromide stained DNA
Lower: hybridization pattern with ³²P-labelled EcoRl-XbaI
        fragment of HSAG-1.

     The clones varied in the extent of the antigenic shifts
they produced but 8 out of 10 of them were capable of
producing the antigen. As these clones were picked
randomly from the 3,400 plaques in the CLL library which
hybridized with the EcoRl-XbaI probe, it follows that our
probe gave us a valid representation of the family of genes
which have the potential to produce this CLL-related
surface antigen. The word "potential" is used because we
believe that most of the HSAG family is not expressed in
the hybrid HCH-1 cells or in human CLL cells; indeed very
few must be expressed in the parental L-73 cells as the
antigen is not even detectable on these cells, a result
which, from other experiments, is not entirely due to
failure of the monoclonal antibody to detect rodent antigen.

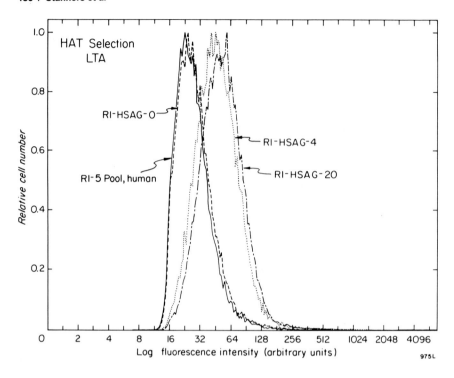

Fig. 5. FACS profiles for fluorescent labelling with monoclonal antibody 37 of the population of L TK$^+$ cells coselected with 200 ng pTK1 (Graham et al., 1980) and 500 ng of cloned human CLL HSAG DNA per 10^6 cells per plate. Note that the abscissa is exponential. "R1-5 Pool human" represents DNA from a pool of control, antigen negative clones. Experimental details are given in Stanners et al. (1981).

The high proportion of expressed clones observed here is presumably due to disruption from their normal location in genomic DNA produced by cloning or perhaps to the artificial nature of the functional test. The mechanism for expression of the HSAG genes in certain malignant cells as opposed to their lack of expression in normal cells is currently under investigation.

This raises a key question: what do these highly repeated genes have to do with malignant transformation? All of the cloned HSAG genes, including the human CLL ones,

Table 2

STRUCTURE OF CLONES WITH HSAG-1 EcoRl-XbaI-LIKE
SEQUENCES FROM HUMAN CLL λ LIBRARY

Clone	EcoRl Fragment Size (kb)	Homology with		Antigen 37 Activity
		EcoRl-XbaI	XbaI-XbaI	
HSAG-0	3.7	+	++	
	3.3		++	−
	3.3	+		
	3.2			
HSAG-20	4.3		+	
	3.3		++	
	2.9	+		+++
	1.9			
HSAG-3	6.0		+/−	
	3.1	+++	+/−	+
	2.7			
HSAG-4	7.8	++	++	+++
	1.65			
HSAG-5	8.0	+++		++
HSAG-6	7.0	++	++	+
	4.1	+/−	++	
HSAG-8	9.2		+/−	+/−
	4.4			
HSAG-10	7.1			
	2.9	++	+/−	−
HSAG-12	5.2			
	4.7		+	+
HSAG-16	6.4	+++	+	+
	3.1			

have the ability to produce morphological transformation
(extreme cell rounding) of L cells, but they do so with a
low efficiency reminiscent of DNA tumor viruses, unlike the
high efficiency of the recently cloned retroviral-like human
oncogenes (Shih & Weinberg, 1982; Goldfarb et al., 1982;
Pulciani et al., 1982). Our current hypothesis is that they
are transposable genetic elements which generate genetic
change and which also code for a surface protein with a
function required for their survival in the genome. In
human lymphoid cell lines they can generate a dominant
malignant change, perhaps by a mechanism analogous to
retroviral LTR gene activation of a gene involved in the
control of cellular proliferation, or by inactivation of a
cis-acting genetic element which suppresses the expression
of such a gene. When applied to mouse fibroblasts in
culture, they can do the same but with the low efficiency
expected of a probabilistic process. This model accommodates
the original observation of a relatively efficient, dominant
malignant transformation of the quasi-normal Chinese hamster
cell line in the cellular hybridization process (Price et al.,
1980), as here the genetic activation of the oncogene would
be in place and conserved during the cell-cell hybridization
process. Thus by emphasizing the antigen during the cloning
process from this hybrid cell we could have cloned the
generator of genetic change rather than the activated
oncogene.

ACKNOWLEDGEMENTS

We thank W.A. Mehring and K. Benzing for technical
assistance and S. Stewart for operation of the FACS. This
work was supported by grants to C.P. Stanners and G.B. Price
from the National Cancer Institute of Canada and from the
Medical Research Council of Canada. J.W. Chamberlain was
supported by the Kenneth M. Hunter Studentship of the
National Cancer Institute of Canada.

Alt FW, Kellems RE, Bertino JR, Schimke RT (1978).
  Selective multiplication of dihydrofolate reductase genes
  in methotrexate-resistant variants of cultured murine
  cells. J Biol Chem 253:1357.
Becker A, Gold M (1975). Isolation of the bacteriophage
  Lambda A-gene protein. Proc Natl Acad Sci USA 72:581.
Benton WD, Davis RW (1977). Screening λgt recombinants
  clones by hybridization to single plaques in situ.
  Science 196:180.

Goldfarb M, Shimigu K, Perucho M, Wigler M (1982).
Isolation and preliminary characterization of a human
transforming gene from T24 bladder carcinoma cells.
Nature 296:404.

Graham FL, Bachetti S, McKinnon R, Stanners CP, Cordell B,
Goodman HM (1980). Transformation of mammalian cells with
DNA using the calcium technique. In Progress in Clinical
and Biological Research: Introduction of Macromolecules
into Viable Mammalian Cells. R. Baserga, C. Croce and
G. Rovera, eds. (New York: Alan R. Liss).

Gusella JF, Keys C, Varsanyi-Breiner A, Kao F-T, Jones C,
Puck TT, Housman D (1980). Isolation and localization of
DNA segments from specific human chromosomes. Proc Natl
Acad Sci USA 77:2829.

Price GB, Sturgeon JFG, Till JE (1980). Focus-forming
ability and surface markers of hamster-human malignant
lymphoma hybrids. Blood 55:351.

Pulciani S, Santos E, Lauver AV, Lang LK, Robbins KC,
Barbacid M (1982). Oncogenes in human tumor cell lines:
Molecular cloning of a transforming gene from human
bladder carcinoma cells. Proc Natl Acad Sci USA 79:2845.

Scheller RH, Anderson DM, Posakony JW, McAllister JB,
Britten RJ, Davidson EH (1981). Repetitive sequences of
the sea urchin genome. II. Subfamily structure and
evolutionary conservation. J Mol Biol 149:15.

Shih C, Weinberg RA (1982). Isolation of a transforming
sequence from a human bladder carcinoma cell line.
Cell 29:161.

Stanners CP, Lam T, Chamberlain JW, Stewart SS, Price GB
(1981). Cloning of a functional gene responsible for the
expression of a cell surface antigen correlated with
human chronic lymphocytic leukemia. Cell 27:211.

Oncogenes and Retroviruses: Evaluation of Basic Findings
and Clinical Potential, pages 185–198

ASP56/LDH$_k$, THE KIRSTEN SARCOMA VIRUS, AND HUMAN CANCER

Garth R. Anderson, Victoria R. Polonis,
Kenneth F. Manly, Raul Saavedra, Mary
Jo Evans and James K. Petell

Roswell Park Memorial Institute
Buffalo, New York 14263

Asp56/LDH$_k$ is an unusual protein which has been detected both enzymatically and as an antigen in diverse
cells transformed by the Kirsten murine sarcoma virus
(Anderson et al. 1979; Anderson et al. 1982). This protein possesses an unusual lactate dehydrogenase activity,
LDH$_k$, distinguished from other isozymes by (i) a highly
cathodic electrophoretic mobility; (ii) reversible inhibition by physiological concentrations of oxygen, (iii)
noncompetitive inhibition by Ap4A, and (iv) a structure of
56,000 dalton subunits, or 35,000 and 22,000 dalton cleavage products (Anderson et al. 1981; Anderson et al.
1982). High levels of an LDH$_k$ activity have also been
found in human cancer tissues, but not in adjoining nontumor tissue (Anderson, Kovacik 1981). We present here
studies on the normal function and regulation of asp56/LDH$_k$,
and data suggesting its possible utility as a serum cancer
marker.

LDH$_k$ as a KiMSV antigen. Initial published results
from our laboratory showed LDH$_k$ as a 35,000 dalton antigen
in KiMSV transformed cells but not in non-rat cells transformed by other agents. Our finding of LDH$_k$ composed of
35,000 and 22,000 dalton subunits (Anderson et al. 1981),
combined with the Scolnick group's finding of a Kirsten
p21 antigen (Scolnick et al. 1979; Shih et al. 1979) could
have been explained if LDH$_k$ were composed of a viral p21
complexed with a cellular p35 component. More recent experiments indicate that this is not the case, and in fact
LDH$_k$ has subunits of 56,000 daltons which can readily be

cleaved to 35,000 and 22,000 dalton fragments (Anderson et al. 1982; JK Petell, unpublished). When LDH_k was purified rapidly from rat muscle or KiMSV infected cells, it was found to be composed of 56,000 dalton subunits.

To help determine whether this 56K form of LDH_k is also associated with KiMSV infection, immune studies analogous to our initial studies in this area have been carried out. Immune studies using rat-specific antisera against anaerobically shocked rat cells had originally identified the 35K and 22K LDH_k antigens in KiMSV transformed cells. Being concerned about proteolysis, we repeated these studies but this time all extracts were stored at -70°. With this procedure, LDH_k as a 56K antigen is seen in KiMSV infected mouse, rat and monkey cells, with no major band at 35K or 22K (Anderson et al. 1982). This antigen is absent in cells transformed by other agents. This 56K antigen comigrated with LDH_k, and LDH_k was an immune competitor of it.

To further evaluate the possibility that the 56K antigen might still be a host protein induced by KiMSV, we have compared by Cleveland gel analysis the 56K antigen from KiMSV transformed NRK (rat) cells with that from KiMSV transformed vero (monkey) cells. These partial proteolytic digests exhibited identical Cleveland gel patterns (Fig. 1), providing additional evidence that the 56K (LDH_k) antigen is virus coded.

Inhibition of LDH_k activity by dipurine nucleoside tetraphosphates. We have published (Anderson et al. 1981) results showing that GTP is a noncompetitive inhibitor of LDH_k; other effective inhibitors were found to be ATP and 5' Gpppp, which was the most effective inhibitor seen in our initial study. Additional studies have since been carried out, examining compounds related to GTP. Two compounds have been found which are far more effective inhibitors of LDH_k activity, namely 5',5'-diguanosine tetraphosphate and 5',5'-diadenosine tetraphosphate (Fig. 2). Diadenosine diphosphate and triphosphate were not effective inhibitors.

On the physiological role of asp56/LDH_k. The inhibition of LDH_k by 5',5'-diadenosine tetraphosphate is intriguing, in that this unusual compound is also implicated in the regulation of DNA synthesis, possibly through associa-

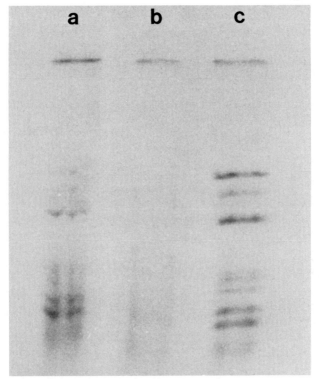

Fig. 1.   Cleveland gel comparisons of asp56/LDH$_k$ from KiMSV
transformed Vero monkey cells with asp56/LDH$_k$ from KiMSV
transformed NRK rat cells, and with p53/SV40 middle-T from
SV40 transformed NRK rat cells. ^{35}S met labeled immune
precipitates described below were electrophoresed on a 10%
SDS polyacrylamide slab gel, and then autoradiographed.
The asp56/LDH$_k$ or p53 bands were then cut from the dried gel
and reelectrophoresed on 10% SDS gels via the Cleveland gel
procedure.   Proteolytic digestion was with 250 ng protease
V-8.   Cleveland gel samples were:
lane (a):   asp56/LDH$_k$ obtained by immune precipitating extracts of ^{35}S met labeled KiMSV-NRK, through use of rabbit
anti asp56 sera.
lane (b):   p53 from rat cells obtained by immune precipitating extracts of ^{35}S met labeled SV40 transformed NRK,
with hamster sera against an anti SV40 inducer tumor.   This
sera was generously provided by M.J. Evans.
lane (c):   asp56/LDH$_k$ obtained by immune precipitating
extracts of ^{35}S met labeled KiMSV-vero, through use of
rabbit anti-asp56 sera.

tion with a 54-57,000 dalton molecular weight polypeptide (Grummt et al. 1979). If asp56/LDH$_k$ were linked to this system, we might predict significant variations in LDH$_k$ activity throughout the cell cycle. Accordingly, we have investigated the expression of LDH$_k$ activity throughout the cell cycle in synchronized cell cultures. As described in Table 1, HeLa cells were found to express minimal LDH$_k$ activity during S phase, but high levels during the rest of the cell cycle. In contrast, expression of other LDH isozymes remained essentially constant throughout the cell cycle. It remains to be determined, however, if the fluctuation seen in LDH$_k$ activity actually represents a link to regulation of DNA synthetic activity.

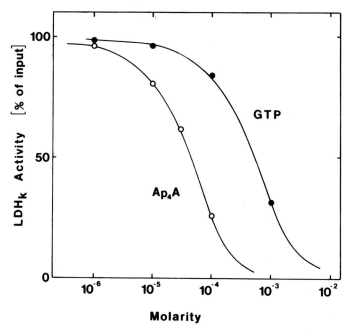

Fig. 2. Inhibition of LDH$_k$ by diadenosine tetraphosphate. Aliquots (10 μg protein) of an S-100 extract of KiMSV infected NRK cells were run on imidazole-borate buffered polyacrylamide slab gels (Anderson et al. 1981) and then individual lanes were activity stained for LDH$_k$ in the presence of Ap4A or GTP. 5 mM NaCN was present in all assay mixes. Activity was quantitated by gel scanning on an integrating densitometer. LDH$_k$ activity is expressed relative to that assayed in the absence of Ap4A or GTP.

Table 1

LDH$_k$ Activity: Variation During the Cell Cycle[a]

Phase of cell cycle	LDH$_{M4}$-LDH$_{H4}$[b]	LDH$_k$[b]
G-1 to S	5	26
S	6.5	1
G-2	6.5	7.5

[a] Suspension cultures of HeLa cells were synchronized by a thymidine block. At two hour intervals following release, parallel samples were assayed for DNA synthesis (^{3}H thymidine incorporation), cell number and LDH isozyme activity. Details of these experiments are presented elsewhere (Evans, Anderson, in preparation).
[b] Activity is reported as densitometer integrator cycles per mg protein. LDH isozymes were quantitated by activity staining of nondenaturing gels which were scanned on an integrating densitometer as described (Anderson et al. 1981). Conventional LDH isozymes (M$_4$, M$_3$H, M$_2$H$_2$, M$_1$H$_3$ and H$_4$) were isolated on tris-glycine buffered gels run anodally. LDH$_k$ was isolated on imidazole-borate buffered gels run cathodally.

Retina represents an unusual tissue in its exhibiting a high level of aerobic glycolysis leading to lactate production, a pattern akin to the metabolism of most cancer tissues (Warburg 1924; Cohen, Noell 1960). We find that LDH$_k$ activity is also expressed at high levels in normal retina (Fig. 3) (Saavedra, Anderson submitted). This is not a reflection of the fact that retina is a neurological tissue; in mammals, brain shows minimal LDH$_k$ activity. In contrast, evolutionary less advanced species (e.g., turtle) show only minor differences between retina and brain (Saavedra et al. in preparation). It should be noted that although retina is metabolically similar to cancer, in retina cells are nonproliferating.

LDH$_k$ activity in human cancer. Cancer tissues from 31 patients (19 carcinomas, 1 sarcoma and 11 leukemias and lymphomas) have been assayed for LDH$_k$ activity. In all but a few cases, adjoining nontumor tissue was also examined for LDH$_k$ activity. As described in detail elsewhere (Anderson, Kovacik 1981), a large majority of carcinomas

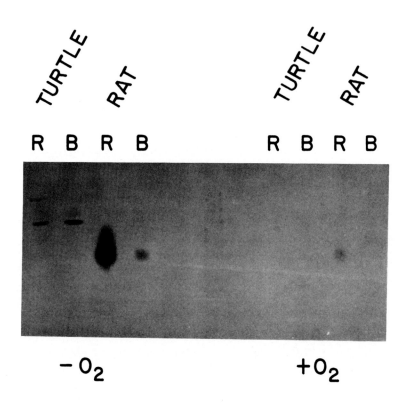

Fig. 3. Asp56/LDH$_k$ in brain and retina tissue of turtle
(Sternotherus odoratus) and rat (Rattus norvegicus).
Brain and retinas were dissected in toto, homogenized and
assayed for asp56/LDH$_k$ activity as described elsewhere
(Anderson et al. 1981). The left-side panel shows a gel
stained for LDH$_k$ activity under anaerobic conditions. R,
retina; B, brain; the right-side panel shows the same as
in left-side panel but stained under aerobic conditions.
Equal amounts (30 μg) of total protein have been loaded on
each well.

showed high levels of LDH$_k$ activity. This observation has
been now extended to the additional tumor types studied.
The specific concentration of LDH$_k$ in a tumor is determined
by assaying aliquots of tumor extract containing increasing
amounts of protein, and determining the amount of LDH$_k$ per
mg of protein. Typical tumor tissue contains 10-100 times
as much LDH$_k$ as does adjoining normal tissue (Fig. 4). As
shown for representative tumors (Fig. 5), there is also a
small elevation seen with other LDH isozymes, but this is
substantially less elevation than that seen with LDH$_k$.
The human tumor LDH$_k$ has been verified as true LDH$_k$ by
the criteria of oxygen responsiveness, inhibition by Ap4A,
and by its highly cathodic electrophoretic mobility.

Since most human tumors were found to express LDH$_k$
activity, we have gone on to examine the sera of cancer
patients in case this enzyme might be of some utility as a
cancer marker. In an initial study, serum from 221 cancer
patients and 30 healthy controls was assayed for LDH$_k$
activity (Polonis 1982; Polonis et al. in preparation).
As summarized in Figure 6, only 2 of the 30 controls (7%)
showed any serum LDH$_k$ and even these were at a low level.
However, over half of the cancer patient sera were found
with significant LDH$_k$ activity. Sera of patients with
metastatic cancer compared with nonmetastatic cancer had a
higher incidence of the enzyme (59% vs. 40%) and when LDH$_k$
was expressed it was seen more often in the highest category. The mean serum LDH$_k$ levels, in gel units per 100 μl
serum, were: healthy controls, 0.5; nonmetastatic cancer
patients, 3.2; and metastatic cancer patients, 7.0. In
studies not shown, there was no correlation between conventional serum LDH level and the level of serum LDH$_k$
(Polonis 1982).

Discussion

Asp56/LDH$_k$ is in itself a most interesting protein,
containing a lactate dehydrogenase activity which is regulated by oxygen and dipurinenucleoside tetraphosphates.
The fact that this protein is expressed in human malignancies adds to its interest. Asp56/LDH$_k$ may also represent
a transforming gene product of the Kirsten sarcoma virus.
We first saw asp56/LDH$_k$ (as cleaved to 35K and 22K polypeptide fragments) in various cells transformed by the Kirsten
sarcoma virus (Anderson et al. 1979; Anderson et al.
1981; Anderson et al. 1982). Evidence that asp56/LDH$_k$ is

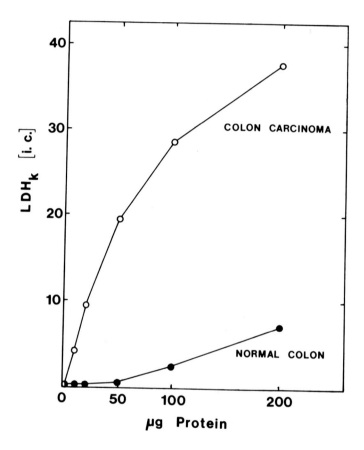

Fig. 4. LDH$_k$ expression in a human colon carcinoma. Extracts were prepared from a human colon carcinoma and from noncancerous adjoining tissue, and assays were carried out using procedures detailed elsewhere (Anderson, Kovacik 1981). LDH$_k$ was determined by electrophoresis on imidazole-borate buffered polyacrylamide gels, followed by activity staining under nitrogen and scanning on an integrating densitometer.

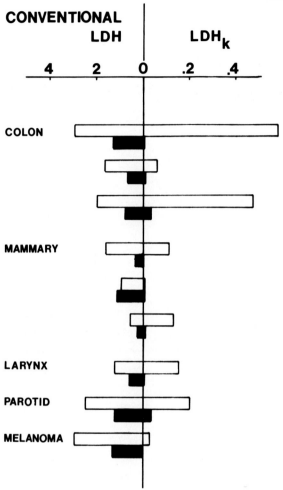

Fig. 5. Expression of conventional LDH and LDH$_k$ in human cancers and adjoining nontumor tissues. S-100 extracts were prepared and analyzed on imidazole-borate gels, as described elsewhere (Anderson, Kovacik 1981). Conventional LDH represents lactate dehydrogenase activity determined spectrophotometrically, in the presence of oxygen, and is expressed as IU/mg. LDH$_k$ was quantitated through assay as in Figure 4, and is expressed as densitometer integrator cycles per microgram of extract protein. 0.2 LDH$_k$ units here is approximately the equivalent of 0.8 IU/mg protein. Cancer tissues (▭); adjoining normal tissues (▬).

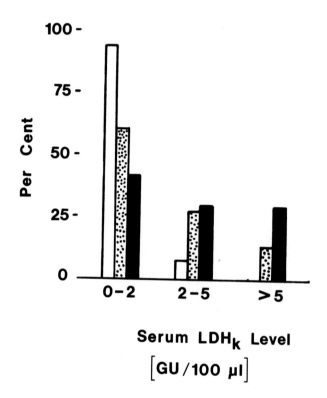

Fig. 6. LDH$_k$ levels in the sera of cancer patients and healthy controls. 100 µl aliquots of serum were analyzed for LDH$_k$ on 3 mm imidazole-borate buffered nondenaturing gels using methods detailed elsewhere (Anderson et al. 1981; Anderson et al. 1982). Activity stained gels were scanned on an integrating densitometer, with activity defined in terms of intetrator units per stained sample. Results were grouped into three categories: negative (0-2); low to moderate (2-5); and high (5). Two hundred fifty-one sera were analyzed, from 30 healthy controls (☐), 124 patients with various nonmetastatic cancers (▨), and 97 patients with metastatic cancers (■).

virus encoded included (i) its detectability (with anti-
rat specific sera) as an antigen in diverse cells (monkey,
mouse, rat, bison) transformed by the Kirsten murine
sarcoma virus, but not in non-rat cells transformed by
other agents; (ii) its expression in uninfected rat cells
induced by anaerobic shock to express RNA homologous to
most (all?) of the rat sequences of the Kirsten sarcoma
virus; and (iii) the fact that LDH$_k$ purified from cells
infected with a temperature sensitive transforming gene
mutant of Kirsten sarcoma virus was thermolabile relative
to LDH$_k$ purified from cells infected with wild type KiMSV.

There is a considerable body of evidence that one
transforming gene product of the Kirsten sarcoma virus is
a 21,000 dalton polypeptide (Ellis et al. 1981; Tsuchida
et al. 1982). This data, obtained in the laboratory of
Scolnick and his collaborators, centers on (i) the finding
of a p21 antigen in Kirsten and Harvey transformed cells,
(ii) the observation that this p21 antigen is apparently
thermolabile as present in ts KiMSV infected cells, (iii)
DNA sequencing data of a clone of ras$_k$, and (iv) the
ability to translate in vitro KiMSV or HaMSV RNA and
obtain the p21. However, the major KiMSV specific in
vitro translation product of KiMSV RNA both in Scolnick's
lab (Shih et al. 1979) and in the lab of DeLeo et al.
(1979) was a polypeptide with a molecular weight of around
53K.

Transfection studies with restriction fragments of
cloned KiMSV DNA have been carried out by both Ellis et
al. (1981) and Norton et al. (1982). Transfectable transforming activity is seen only with a large restriction
fragment. The smallest reported piece with transfectable
transforming activity is a fragment starting at the 5' LTR
and continuing for 3.1 kb. Studies with deletion mutants
of KiMSV have defined ca 1.5 kb which are not nonessential
for transformation (Tsuchida et al. 1982), an amount con-
siderably larger than required to encode p21.

Especially in view of the fact that Kirsten homologous
onc genes are found in human cancer (Der et al. 1982), two
key issues exist regarding the relationship of asp56/LDH$_k$
to the Kirsten sarcoma virus. First, is asp56/LDH$_k$
actually encoded by Kirsten sequences, and second, if so,
does it in fact represent a transforming gene product?
The results from Scolnick's lab are not necessarily

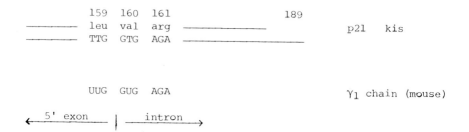

Fig. 7. Sequences homologous to a known 9 base RNA splice junction signal are present in the region of the Kirsten sarcoma virus encoding p21 kis. The sequence data for the p21 coding region is from Tsuchida et al. (1982). The γ1 chain splice junction sequence is from Honjo (1979). It should be pointed out that other 9 base splice junction sequences are known but are closely related to the γ1 sequence shown (Lerner et al. 1980).

incompatible with our observations suggesting asp56/LDH$_k$ is encoded by the KiMSV transforming gene. One possibility is that we may be dealing with an overlapping gene situation akin to the small t/large T of SV40, where p21 would be made from a different spliced messenger than asp56/LDH$_k$. If this were the case, one would expect to find a RNA splice junction signal in the sequences encoding p21. In fact, a known 9-base RNA splice signal does exist at the bases encoding amino acids 159 to 161 of the Kirsten p21 kis transforming protein (Fig. 7). If this splice junction signal is in fact used, an additional larger polypeptide containing the first 159 amino acids of p21 would also be synthesized. A second possibility is that asp56/LDH$_k$ is encoded by KiMSV genes but is not essential for transformation. Finally, in the absence of in vitro translation studies, it remains conceivable that asp56/LDH$_k$ is a highly conserved host gene product specifically induced upon transformation by KiMSV. However, this last possibility would be most difficult to reconcile with the immunological and thermolability data we have obtained. Understanding the significance of LDH$_k$ expression in human cancer demands a concrete determination of whether LDH$_k$ is truly a virus onc gene product. These studies are now in progress.

Acknowledgements

We wish to thank William Kovacik, Becky K. Farkas, Clara Cordoba and Victoria Onorato for valuable technical assistance. We also thank Joel Huberman for pointing out Ap4A to us, and George Todaro for initially suggesting we pursue the serum marker possibilities of LDH_k. This work was supported by funding from the Muscular Dystrophy Association, the Sklarow Foundation, and grant CA32022 from the NIH.

References

Anderson GR, Kovacik WP (1981). LDH_k, an unusual oxygen-sensitive lactate dehydrogenase expressed in human cancer. Proc Natl Acad Sci USA 78:3209-3213.

Anderson GR, Kovacik WP, Marotti KR (1981). LDH_k, a uniquely regulated cryptic lactate dehydrogenase associated with transformation by the Kirsten murine sarcoma virus. J Biol Chem 256:10583-10591.

Anderson GR, Marotti KR, Whitaker-Dowling PA (1979). A candidate rat-specific gene product of the Kirsten murine sarcoma virus. Virology 99:31-48.

Anderson GR, Polonis VR, Petell JK, Saavedra RA, Manly KF, Matovcik LM (1982). $Asp56/LDH_k$ in human cancer. In Whitt G (ed): "Isozymes", Vol 7, Allan R Liss, NY in press.

Cohen LH, Noell WK (1960). Glucose catabolism of rabbit retina before and after development of visual function. J Neurochem 5:253-276.

DeLeo AB, Jay G, Appella E, Dubois GC, Law LW, Old LJ (1970). Detection of a transformation-related antigen in transformed cells of the mouse. Proc Natl Acad Sci USA 76:2420-2424.

Der CJ, Krontiris TG, Cooper GM (1982). Transforming genes of human bladder and lung carcinoma are homologous to the ras genes. Proc Natl Acad Sci USA 79:3637-3640.

Ellis RW, DeFeo D, Maryak JM, Young HA, Shih TY, Chang EH, Lowy DR, Scolnick EM (1980). Dual evolutionary origin for the rat genetic sequences of Harvey mouse sarcoma virus. J Virol 36:408-420.

Grummt F, Waltl G, Jantzen HM, Hamprecht K, Heubscher U, Kuenzle C (1979). Diadenosine 5',5'-tetraphosphate, a ligand of the 57 kd subunit of DNA polymerase α. Proc Natl Acad Sci USA 76:6081-6085.

Honjo T, Obata M, Yamawaki Y, Kataoka T, Kawakami T, Takahashi N, Moro Y (1979). Cloning and complete nucleotide sequence of mouse immunoglobin γ1 chain gene. Cell 18:559-568.

Lerner MR, Bogle JA, Mount SM, Wolin SL, Steitz JA (1980). Are snRNPs involved in splicing? Nature 283:220-224.

Norton JD, Carter AT, Avery RJ (1982). Restriction endonuclease mapping of unintegrated proviral DNA of Kirsten murine sarcoma virus. J Gen Virol 58:95-106.

Polonis VR (1982). A quantitative analysis of LDH_k, an unusual isozyme of lactate dehydrogenase, in serum of cancer patients. M.S. thesis, Niagara University.

Scolnick EM, Papageorge AG, Shih TY (1979). Guanine nucleotide binding activity as an assay for src protein of rat derived murine sarcoma viruses. Proc Natl Acad Sci USA 76:5355-5359.

Shih TY, Weeks MO, Young HA, Scolnick EM (1979). p21 of Kirsten sarcoma virus is thermolabile in a viral mutant temperature sensitive for the maintenance of transformation. J Virol 31:546-556.

Shih TY, Weeks MO, Young HA, Scolnick EM (1979). Identification of the sarcoma virus-coded phosphoprotein in nonproducer cells transformed by Kirsten or Harvey murine sarcoma virus. Virology 96:64-79.

Tsuchida N, Ryder T, Ohtsubo E (1982). Nucleotide sequence of the oncogene encoding the p21 transforming protein of KiMSV. Science 217:937-938.

Warburg O, Posener K, Negalein E (1924). Metabolism of carcinoma cells. Biochem Z 152:309-344.

Oncogenes and Retroviruses: Evaluation of Basic Findings
and Clinical Potential, pages 199–205
© 1983 Alan R. Liss, Inc., 150 Fifth Avenue, New York, NY 10011

THE SEROLOGICAL ANALYSIS OF HUMAN CANCER.   IDENTIFICATION OF
DIFFERENTIATION ANTIGENS ON MELANOMA AND MELANOCYTES.

Alan N. Houghton, M.D.

Memorial Sloan-Kettering Cancer Center
1275 York Avenue
New York, New York   10021

With the advent of the hybridoma technology, the
resolving power of serology to study cancer antigens has
increased by orders of magnitude, and this has led to a
resurgence of investigations of human cancer antigens. As
such, monoclonal antibodies can be powerful tools to study
the products or by-products of genes which are involved in
malignant transformation. This paper is concerned with the
use of serological probes in the analysis of human cancer,
in particular, with our studies of malignant melanoma.

These studies have focused on the identification and
characterization of differentiation antigens on melanoma
cells by mouse monoclonal antibodies. Differentiation
antigens are antigens that distinguish cells in distinct
pathways of differentiation, for instance distinguish
lymphocytes from hepatocytes, or antigens that distinguish
cells at different stages of differentiation in the same
pathway, for instance distinguish an early thymocyte from a
mature T cell (Boyse and Old, 1969). A second question which
can be studied with serological probes is whether cells undergo antigenic changes during malignant transformation which
are recognized by the host's immune system. The appearance
of antigens may be due to quantitative changes in gene expression, or antigens may appear *de novo*, in the instance of
transformation-specific or tumor-specific antigens. The
recent developments in the human monoclonal antibody technology permit a new and broad approach to this second problem.

Our studies of mouse monoclonal antibodies to melanoma
cell surface antigens started as an attempt to map surface

antigens of melanoma cells, in particular, searching for
antibodies to tumor-restricted antigens (Dippold *et al.*,
1980). To date, 50 cell surface antigens of melanoma have
been defined by our group. Twenty of these antigens were
found to be broadly distributed on most cell types, 17
showed intermediate distribution and 13 were restricted to
malignant melanoma and closely related cell types.

Two things became clear from these studies. First,
none of these antigens were tumor-restricted; even the most
restricted antigens were also present on normal melanocytes.
The other point is that the majority of antigens were
expressed on only a proportion of melanomas, dividing melanoma cell lines into distinguishable subsets. Some antigens,
such as the antigen R_{24}, were found on virtually all melanomas, and as such may be markers of neuroectoderm differentiation. Other antigens were expressed only on a small
proportion of melanomas. This diversity of antigen expression on melanomas suggested a corresponding diversity
of antigenic phenotype of normal cells in the melanocyte
differentiation pathway. To pursue this idea, the surface
antigens of normal melanocytes and a panel of melanoma cell
lines were analyzed (Houghton *et al.*, 1982).

Cutaneous melanocytes are pigmented cells located at
the junction between the dermis and epidermis. Melanoma
of the skin arises from melanocytes or one of its precur-
sors. Melanocytes comprise only a small fraction of the
cells in the skin, and therefore have not been easy to isolate, but recently a method has been developed to grow
relatively pure populations of melanocytes in tissue culture
(Eisinger and Marko, 1982). Melanocytes have two easily
recognizable differentiated properties. First, they are
able to synthesize the pigment melanin using the specialized
cellular enzyme, tyrosinase. Secondly, mature melanocytes
have dendritic processes which donate pigment to the
surrounding keratinocytes, hence imbuing the skin with color.
In culture, fetal and newborn melanocytes grow as bipolar,
spindle-shaped cells. Melanocytes of adult skin show more
differentiated properties, with a polydendritic morphology
and heavy pigmentation.

Fetal, newborn and adult melanocytes were tested using
a panel of monoclonal antibodies directed against 37 melanoma cell surface antigens. Melanoma antigens can be grouped into four categories on the basis of their expression on

melanocytes. First are those not detected on fetal, newborn or adult melanocytes. These antigens are expressed by a proportion of melanoma cell lines. A second group of antigens are those expressed on fetal and newborn melanocytes but not adult. A third category of antigens are detected on adult but not newborn melanocytes, and the largest group of antigens are detected on fetal, newborn and adult melanocytes.

On the basis of antigen expression on fetal, newborn and adult melanocytes, we have identified antigens which appear to be early, intermediate or late markers of melanocyte differentiation (Table 1). Early markers, M-2, M-3 and HLA-DR, are found on some melanomas, but are not detected on fetal, newborn or adult melanocytes. Intermediate markers are found on fetal and newborn melanocytes, but not adult (M-4, M-6 and M-7). Late markers are found on adult melanocytes, but not fetal or newborn (M-9 and M-10).

Table 1

CELL SURFACE ANTIGENS OF MELANOCYTE DIFFERENTIATION

	Fetal/Newborn Melanocytes	Adult Melanocytes	Melanoma
Early Markers			
M-2			
M-3	−	−	+ or −
HLA-DR			
Intermediate Markers			
M-4			
M-5	+	−	+ or −
M-6			
Late Markers			
M-9	−	+	+ or −
M-10			

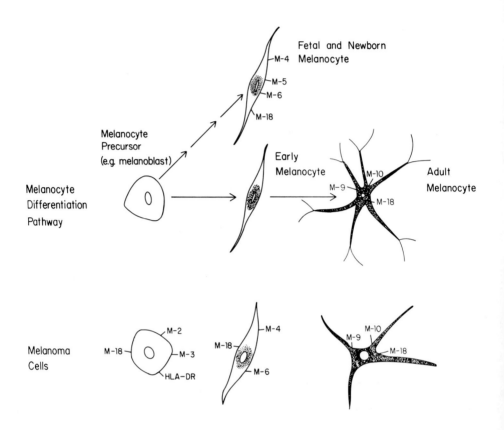

FIG. 1. Proposed pathway of melanocyte differentiation based
on surface antigenic phenotype and morphology. The phenotype
of melanomas corresponding to early, intermediate or late
stages in the melanocyte pathway is also shown. M-18 antigen
is found on all stages of melanocyte differentiation and is
present on all melanoma cells.

When these eight systems were used to type melanoma cell lines, it was found that melanomas could be grouped into three general categories on the basis of expression of early, intermediate and late melanocyte markers. When melanomas were ordered according to their antigenic expression, early or late, there was a correlation between antigen phenotype and other differentiation characteristics, including morphology, pigmentation and tyrosinase activity. Melanomas expressing early markers, such as M-2, M-3 and HLA-DR usually have an epithelial morphology, lack pigmentation and have no tyrosinase activity. In contrast, melanomas expressing late markers have a spindle or dendritic shape, are pigmented and can have high levels of tyrosinase activity. The interpretation we draw from this data is that the phenotype of melanoma cells resembles the phenotype of normal cells in the melanocyte lineage.

Thus, we have proposed a rudimentary map of the melanocyte lineage (Figure 1). Although the normal melanocyte precursor, or melanoblast, has not been clearly identified, its phenotype has been inferred from melanomas expressing early differentiation markers, and monoclonal antibodies to these early markers should be useful in the physical isolation of the melanoblast. These studies suggest two interpretations for the pathogenesis of melanoma. Melanomas could arise at any one of a number of stages in the melanocyte lineage with the differentiated phenotype then relatively frozen. Alternatively, malignant transformation could occur at a preferential stage, for instance transformation occurring early in the melanocyte pathway, in a progenitor cell, with the transformed cells then undergoing varying degrees of differentiation. In favor of the capacity of melanoma cells to differentiate is the phenotypic heterogeneity of tumor cells in melanoma metastases. Certainly, pathologists have long noted that melanoma cells in a lesion may have different shapes and degrees of pigmentation. In studies of antigen expression on frozen tissue sections of melanoma using indirect immunofluorescence techniques, we have found striking differences in antigen expression of melanoma metastases. Heterogeneity of the expression of the early differentiation antigen, HLA-DR, and the intermediate melanocyte antigen, M-4, within a single lesion has been a very common characteristic of lesions from more than 50 melanoma patients studied to date. These observations are more consistent with a model of early stage transformation and variable capacity to differentiate. This matter of the stage of transformation may be clarified by further studies, including our current attempts to transform melanocytes from different stages of differentiation.

Having discussed what is known about melanoma antigens that the mouse recognizes, it is appropriate to turn briefly to the question of what melanoma antigens to humans recognize. The most direct approach to this question to date has come from studies using autologous combinations of tumor cells and sera from the same patient (Carey *et al.*, 1976; Shiku *et al.*, 1976; Shiku *et al.*, 1977; and Albino *et al.*, 1981). This system of autologous typing has eliminated reactions to allogeneic surface antigens which have so often confounded serological studies. More directly, it has provided evidence for humoral immunity of cancer patients to their own tumor.

In this way, three classes of surface antigens were defined on melanoma. Class 1 antigens are unique; their expression is restricted only to the autologous tumor cell, and they are not found on melanomas from other individuals. These antigens remain candidates for tumor-specific antigens. Class 2 antigens are shared tumor antigens, found on autologous and allogeneic melanoma cells as well as some normal neuroectodermal cells, while Class 3 antigens are widely distributed on malignant and normal cells. To date, of the 130 patients studied, 7 melanoma patients have been identified with antibodies to the Class 1 antigens and 5 patients with antibodies to the Class 2 antigens.

An exciting new approach to the problem of immune recognition has been the application of the hybridoma technology to the production of human monoclonal antibodies. The expectation is that new tumor antigens will be identified and that this method will go beyond autologous typing. In particular, the specificity of lymphocytes in lymph nodes around the tumor, as well as lymphocytes infiltrating the tumor itself, can now be studied. Perhaps analysis of human cancer antigens by human monoclonal antibodies will lead back to differentiation antigens. However, the critical question for human monoclonal antibodies, and cancer immunology, remains. Do antigenic changes occur during malignant transformation which are recognized by the host's immune system?

Albino AP, Lloyd KO, Houghton AN, Oettgen HF, Old LJ (1981). Heterogeneity in surface antigen expression and glycoprotein expression of cell lines derived from different metastases of the same patient. J Exp Med 154:1764.

Boyse EA, Old LJ (1969). Some aspects of normal and abnormal cell surface antigens. Ann Rev Genet 3:269.

Carey TE, Takahashi T, Resnick LA, Oettgen HF, Old LJ (1976). Cell surface antigens of human malignant melanoma. I. Mixed hemadsorption assay for humoral immunity to cultured autologous melanoma cells. Proc Natl Acad Sci USA 73:3278.

Dippold WG, Lloyd KO, Li LTC, Ikeda H, Oettgen HF, Old LJ (1980). Cell surface antigens of human malignant melanoma. Definition of six new antigenic systems with mouse monoclonal antibodies. Proc Natl Acad Sci USA 77:6114.

Eisinger M, Marko O (1982). Selective proliferation of normal human melanocytes *in vitro* in the presence of phorbol ester and cholera toxin. Proc Natl Acad Sci USA 79:2018.

Houghton AN, Eisinger M, Albino AP, Cairncross JG, Old LJ (1982). Surface antigens of melanocytes and melanomas. Markers for melanocyte differentiation and melanoma subsets. J Exp Med (submitted).

Shiku H, Takahashi T, Oettgen HF, Old LJ (1976). Cell surface antigens of human malignant melanoma. II. Serological typing with immune adherence assays and definition of two new surface antigens. J Exp Med 144:873.

Shiku H, Takahashi T, Resnick LA, Oettgen HF, Old LJ (1977). Cell surface antigens of human malignant melanoma. III. Recognition of autoantibodies with unusual characteristics. J Exp Med 145:784.

Oncogenes and Retroviruses: Evaluation of Basic Findings
and Clinical Potential, pages 207–222
© 1983 Alan R. Liss, Inc., 150 Fifth Avenue, New York, NY 10011

RETROVIRAL onc GENES IN HUMAN NEOPLASIA

Stuart A. Aaronson, Claire Y. Dunn,
Nelson W. Ellmore, Alessandra Eva

Laboratory of Cellular and Molecular Biology,
National Cancer Institute, Bethesda, MD 20205

Type-C retroviruses consist of chronic and acute transforming retroviruses. The chronic viruses when inoculated
into susceptible animals cause tumors, mostly leukemias, but
only after a latent period of several months. These viruses
replicate in the absence of any apparent transforming effect
on known assay cells in tissue culture. In contrast, acute
transforming viruses induce tumors within a very short
period of days to weeks. They cause a variety of tumors,
including sarcomas, hematopoietic tumors, and even carcinomas.
In tissue culture, these viruses generally induce foci of
transformation in appropriate assay cells.

Over the past two decades, many scientists have turned
their attention to the study of these viruses in efforts to
learn more about how normal cells become malignant. While
years ago one could not predict how soon or how great the
rewards of this approach would be, we are now seeing its
fruits in studies that are ever more directly applicable to
man.

The retrovirus genome. The chronic leukemia virus
genome contains gag, pol and env genes, which code for internal structural proteins, reverse transcriptase, and envelope
proteins, respectively (Baltimore 1974). The proviral genome
also contains a repeat sequence of anywhere from 300-600
bases at either terminus of the viral genome (Fig. 1).
These long terminal repeats (LTRs) contain signals for the
initiation and termination of transcription and resemble
prokaryotic transposable elements (Dhar et al. 1980;
Shimotohno et al. 1980). Chronic leukemia viruses do not

appear to possess an additional discrete transforming gene
and the mechanism of transformation by these agents is not
as yet resolved.

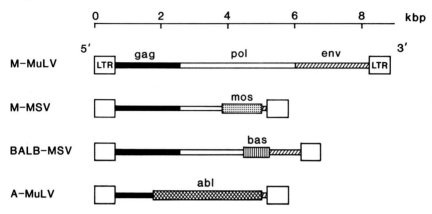

Fig. 1. Relationship of three murine transforming retroviral
genomes to the chronic leukemia virus genome. The onc gene
of each retrovirus is indicated by a differently shaded box
to denote the different cellular origin of each. Each of
the viral genomes was cloned and physically characterized as
previously reported (Tronick et al. 1979; Srinivasan et al.
1981; Andersen et al. 1981.)

The mode of action of acute transforming viruses is
somewhat better understood and has become immediately relevant to understanding of naturally occurring malignancies.
Our ability to learn about these viruses has been immeasur-
ably aided by the development and application of modern
molecular biological techniques. It is apparent from
observation of the physical maps (Fig. 1) of three mouse
derived acute transforming retroviruses molecularly cloned
in our laboratory (Andersen et al. 1981; Srinivasan et al.
1981; Tronick et al. 1979) why years ago we initially found
that these viruses were capable of transformation but were
replication defective (Aaronson, Rowe 1970). In each case,
the genome of the acute transforming virus is smaller than
that of the chronic leukemia virus. In addition, each has
substituted a discrete segment of information. Thus, each
of these viruses lacks essential leukemia virus information
required for its replication.

Of particular importance with respect to cancer research are discrete segments which are unrelated to the leukemia virus genome. In the viruses shown, each of these segments differs from the other; however, when DNA probes are prepared from these segments, they detect in normal mouse cell DNA not multiple, but one or at most a few copies of related sequences. Similar findings by a number of laboratories have led to the understanding that acute transforming retroviruses have arisen in nature by recombination of leukemia viruses with cellular genes.

Retroviral onc genes. The cell-derived onc genes of transforming retroviruses are required for viral transforming functions. This was initially demonstrated by classic genetic approaches with Rous sarcoma virus, one of the few transforming viruses which possesses both transforming and replication functions. Transformation-defective mutants are spontaneously generated at relatively high frequency, and these mutants were shown to have specifically deleted the cell-derived src gene (for review see Bishop 1978 and Wang 1978).

An independent approach has utilized deletion analysis of replication-defective transforming retroviral DNAs. This approach can be illustrated by a molecular genetic analysis of the cloned DNA of simian sarcoma virus (SSV), a primate derived acute transforming virus. In order to localize the region of SSV required for transformation, we constructed a variety of deletion mutants from a molecular clone of SSV DNA and tested their ability to transform NIH/3T3 cells in a transfection assay (Robbins et al. in press). As shown in Fig. 2, the intact viral genome (pSSV-11) exhibited a transforming activity of $10^{4.1}$ focus-forming units/pmol viral DNA. A subgenomic clone, pSSV 3/1, from which the 3' long terminal repeat (LTR) was deleted, showed no reduction in biologic activity. In contrast, pSSV 3/2, a subclone lacking the 3' LTR as well as all but 25 bp of v-sis, demonstrated no detectable transforming activity. These results strongly imply the essential nature of v-sis in SSV transformation.

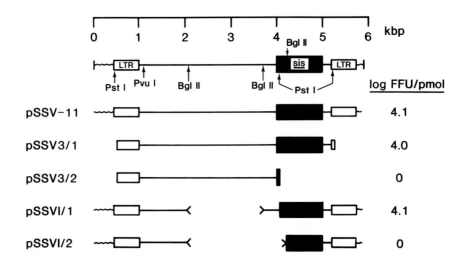

Fig. 2. Construction and biologic analysis of SSV deletion mutants. The integrated form of SSV was excised from λ-SSV-11 Cl 1 (Robbins et al. in press) and purified by elution from a preparative agarose gel. pSSV 3/1 and 2 were constructed by cloning products of a reaction in which purified SSV DNA was partially digested with PstI. pSSV-11 was obtained by cloning the λ-SSV-11 Cl 1 insert at the EcoRI site of pBR322. pSSV I/1 and 2 were constructed by limited BglII digestion of pSSV-11 followed by religation. In each case, the structure of individual deletion mutants was determined by restriction enzyme and Southern blotting analysis. Transfection of NIH/3T3 cells with plasmids containing SSV wt or mutant DNAs was performed by the calcium phosphate precipitation technique (Graham, van der Eb, 1973). Transformed foci were scored at 14-21 days.

pSSV I/1, a mutant lacking an internal 1.8-kbp BglII fragment (Fig. 2), transformed NIH/3T3 cells with an efficiency of $10^{4.1}$ ffu/pmol viral DNA. However, a subclone, pSSV I/2, which lacked an additional stretch of 245 bp of SSAV sequences as well as the first 339 bp of v-sis, possessed no transforming activity. These results localize the SSV transforming gene to a region encompassing v-sis, along with 254 and 302 bp of flanking SSAV sequences, to the left and right of v-sis, respectively (Robbins et al. in press). These and analogous studies with other trans-

forming retroviral DNAs have documented that their onc genes
are responsible for the induction and maintenance of the
virus transformed state.

The number of onc genes incorporated by retroviruses
is limited. Analysis of independent isolates of transforming
retroviruses has indicated that there are a limited number
of distinct cellular onc sequences with transforming potential
that such viruses have transduced. Of more than 20 independent transforming retrovirus isolates, certain isolates of
the same species appear to contain the same or closely
related onc genes (Stehelin et al. 1976; Donoghue et al. 1979;
Duesberg, Vogt 1979; Frankel et al. 1979; Ellis et al. 1981;
Ghysdael et al. 1981; Andersen et al. 1981). Furthermore,
relatedness has been demonstrated between sarcoma virus-
specific sequences of transforming viruses obtained from
species as diverse as chicken and cat (Shibuya et al. 1980;
Barbacid et al. 1981; Beemon 1981). These findings have
emerged from studies utilizing sarcoma virus-specific cDNA
probes or antibodies capable of recognizing immunologically
related sarcoma viral gene products.

When we compared the molecularly cloned onc gene (v-bas)
of BALB-MSV, a spontaneous mouse sarcoma virus isolate, with
the ras gene of rat-derived Harvey-MSV genome, a colinear
750-bp region of homology was observed (Fig. 3). Moreover,
BALB-MSV transformants were found to express high levels of
a 21,000 dalton protein, immunologically related to the ras
gene product, p21 (Andersen et al. 1981). Thus, bas and ras
represent retroviral transforming gene homologs that were
independently transduced by mouse type C viruses from the
genomes of rat and mouse species (Andersen et al. 1981.)

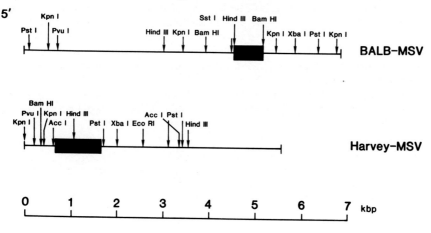

Comparison of the molecular structures of BALB-MSV and Harvey-MSV (Fig. 3) reveals that their onc genes are in very different locations. Whereas Harvey-MSV ras is near the 5' terminus of the genome, BALB-MSV bas is located toward the 3' end of the molecule. Ra-MSV is an independent rat-derived transforming virus isolate (Rasheed et al. 1978), which contains ras sequences (Young et al. 1979). Its transforming gene product is synthesized as a larger polypeptide comprised of rat helper viral gag and p21 products (Young et al. 1981). This suggests that its gene sequence organization is different from that of either BALB- or Harvey-MSV. Thus, whatever function(s) helper viral sequences provide for replication and expression of this transforming gene, the gene can be localized with the viral genome in very different positions.

There is emerging evidence that onc genes incorporated by retroviruses may comprise an even smaller number of families of evolutionarily related genes. Kirsten-MSV codes for a transforming protein immunologically related to those of BALB- and Harvey-MSV despite the fact that its onc sequences originate from a different cellular gene (Ellis et al. 1981.)

While there is little detectable nucleotide sequence homology between Kirsten-MSV ras and the onc genes of either BALB- or Harvey-MSV, nucleotide sequence analysis of these genes has revealed striking homology at the protein level (Dhar et al. 1982; Tsuchida et al. 1982; Reddy et al. unpublished observations). Such homology is likely to have resulted from divergence from a common ancestral gene, although convergent evolution cannot be excluded. Similarly, src, Moloney-MSV mos, and the onc gene from an avian trans-forming retrovirus, Y73, lack detectable relatedness by molecular hybridization and possess extensive homology with different cellular genes. However, these onc genes demon-strate varying degrees of homology at the nucleotide sequence level (Van Beveren et al. 1981; Kitamura et al. 1982). Thus, acute transforming viruses have incorporated from a potential battery of thousands of cellular genes only a very

---

Fig. 3. Physical maps of the BALB-MSV and Harvey-MSV DNAs. The positions of bas and ras sequences are indicated by heavy lines.

few. These findings strongly argue that the number of
cellular genes that can be altered or activated to become
transforming genes when incorporated within the retrovirus
genome is limited.

    Onc gene products. Retroviral onc genes appear to act
by means of translational products. In so..e cases, it has
been possible to detect such proteins by means of antisera
prepared in animals bearing tumors induced by these viruses.
Using such antisera, the Rous sarcoma virus src gene product
has been shown to be a protein kinase (Collet, Erickson
1978; Levinson et al. 1978) with rather unique specificity
for phosphorylating tyrosine residues (Hunter, Sefton
1980). Analogous functions have been ascribed to the onc
genes of several other viruses.

    We have utilized another strategy to obtain antisera
capable of recognizing onc gene products. Due to the
advances of recombinant DNA and nucleotide sequencing, it is
possible to prepare antisera to peptides synthesized on the
basis of a known nucleotide sequence. By such an approach,
it is hoped that the antiserum will be capable of recognizing
the entire translational product of the gene in question.

    The simian sarcoma virus sis gene, as well as several
other onc genes sequenced by scientists in our laboratory,
contain open reading frames that initiate in helper viral
sequences within a few bases to the left of their cell-
derived onc gene and continue for several hundred nucleotides
into the onc genes themselves (Devare et al. 1982; Reddy et
al. 1981; Reddy et al. in preparation). A peptide comprised
of 15 amino acids from the N-terminal region of the predicted
sis protein was used to immunize rabbits. As shown in
Figure 4, this antiserum detected a 28,000 MW protein in
SSV-transformed cells that could not be precipitated with
preimmune serum nor detected by the antiserum in uninfected
cells. Moreover, precipitation of this protein could be
completely inhibited by preincubation with the peptide
(Fig. 4; Robbins et al. in press).

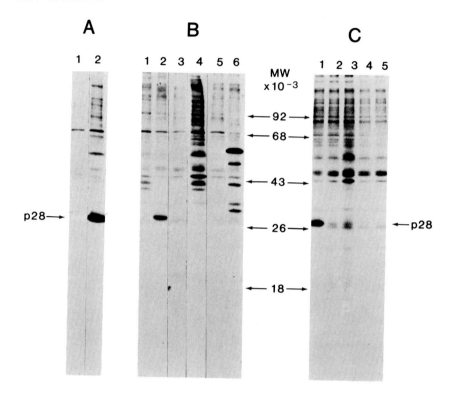

Fig. 4. <u>In vivo</u> detection of a v-<u>sis</u> translational product
by immunoprecipitation analysis (Robbins et al. in press).
Subconfluent cultures (around 10^7 cells per 10 cm petri
dish) were labeled for 3 h at 37˚C with 4 ml of methionine-
free Dulbecco's modified Eagle's minimal essential medium
containing 100 µCi [^{35}S]-methionine (1,200 Ci/nmol,
Amersham) per ml. Radiolabeled cells were lysed with 1 ml
of a buffer containing 10 mM sodium phosphate, pH 7.5, 100
mM NaCl, 1% Triton X-10, 0.5% sodium deoxycholate and 0.1 mM
phenylmethyl-sulfonyl fluoride per Petri dish, clarified
at 100,000 xg for 30 min, and divided into four identical
aliquots. Each aliquot was incubated with 4 µl of antisera
for 60 min at 4˚C. Immunoprecipitates were recovered with
the aid of <u>Staphylococcus aureus</u> protein A bound to sepharose
beads (Pharmacia) and analyzed by electrophoresis in sodium
dodecyl sulfate - 14% polyacrylamide gels as described
(Robbins et al. in press). (A) Immunoprecipitation of
labeled extracts of SSV (SSAV)-transformed producer (lane 1)
or uninfected (lane 2) marmoset cells with anti-SSV <u>sis</u>

This protein corresponds in size to that predicted for the SSV transforming protein from our sequence studies (Devare et al. 1982), further indicating that we have indeed identified the SSV transforming gene product in SSV-transformed cells. Hopefully, this approach will be useful not only in characterizing this protein but will help as well in identifying and characterizing the onc gene products of other acute transforming retroviruses.

Chromosomal mapping of human onc gene homologues. Genes related to retroviral onc genes are well conserved in human DNA. It is possible to map these genes to specific human chromosomes by testing for the presence of human DNA fragments related to a specific onc gene in somatic cell hybrids possessing varying numbers of human chromosomes as well as in segregants of such hybrids. By this approach, sis has been assigned to chromosome 22 (Swan et al. 1982), while mos has been mapped to chromosome 8 (Prakash et al. 1982). The chromosomal assignments of additional onc genes indicate that such genes are distributed throughout the human genome (Dalla-Favera et al. 1982).

The chromosomes to which sis and mos have been assigned are known to exhibit highly reproducible translocations in chronic myelogenous leukemia (Rowley 1980) and Burkitt's lymphoma (Bernheim et al. 1981), respectively. Klein (1981) has speculated that chromosomal translocations may result in the activation of onc genes. Studies are currently in progress to resolve whether the specific activation of onc genes by such a mechanism plays a role in these tumors.

Human onc gene homologues are transcribed in human tumor cells. We sought to determine whether the human

---

peptide serum. (B) Immunoprecipitation of labeled extracts of SSV clone 11 transformed nonproducer NRK cells with pre-immune rabbit serum (lane 1), anti-sis peptide serum (lane 2) or anti-SSAV serum (lane 6). Anti-sis peptide serum was also used to immunoprecipitate uninfected (lane 3) Moloney murine sarcoma virus-transformed nonproducer (lane 4) or SSAV-infected (lane 5) NRK cell extracts. (C) Immunoprecipitation of extracts of SSV clone 11 transformed nonproducer NRK cells with anti-sis peptide serum which was preincubated with 0, 0.1, 0.3, 1 or 10 µg (lanes 1-5, respectively) of sis peptide.

homologues of retroviral onc genes are transcribed in human
cells and whether their expression could be in some way
correlated with the malignant state (Eva et al. 1982; Westin
et al. 1982). We analyzed polyadenylated RNAs from a large
series of tumor cells derived from different solid tumors
and hematopoietic malignancies. The onc genes of transforming retroviruses known to induce tumors of a wide
variety of tissue types were utilized as probes. There was
rather striking specificity in the detection of transcripts
related to certain onc genes such as that of simian sarcoma
virus (Eva et al. 1982; Westin et al. 1982).

Sis related transcripts were found only in certain
fibrosarcoma or glioblastoma cells but not in normal fibroblasts, other solid tumors, or for the most part in any
normal or malignant hematopoietic cells analyzed. In contrast,
we found that certain onc genes detected related transcripts
not only in tumor cells but in normal cells as well (Eva et
al. 1982; Westin et al. 1982). Whatever their role in tumors,
these genes were likely to be functioning and thus important
in human cells.

Isolation of human oncogenes by DNA-mediated gene
transfer. An independent approach to the identification of
transforming genes has come from the application of DNA-
mediated gene transfer techniques. DNAs of a variety of
tumors, including some of human origin, have been shown to
induce foci of transformation upon transfection of suitable
assay cells (Cooper 1982). Several such dominant transforming
genes have been isolated by molecular cloning techniques.
The first oncogene of human origin has been isolated from EJ
and T24 human bladder carcinoma cells (Goldfarb et al. 1982;
Pulciani et al. 1982; Shih, Weinberg 1982).

The number of oncogenes detected by transfection analysis
appears to be limited. For example, different mammary carcinomas appear to possess the same activated cellular sequences,
whereas many lung and colon carcinomas possess a different
oncogene (Cooper 1982).

Relationship of human oncogenes to retroviral onc genes.
It was of interest to ascertain whether any of the newly
identified human oncogenes were related to the set of transforming genes that have been transduced by retroviruses. We
observed that the T24 human bladder tumor gene reciprocally
hybridized to v-bas, the onc gene of BALB-MSV. A cloned

6.6-kbp BamHI human DNA fragment harboring the T24 oncogene
was readily hybridized with a DNA probe containing 675 bp of
v-bas, the onc gene of BALB-MSV. Morevoer, v-bas DNA was
detected with a probe composed of the T24 oncogene. Additional studies localized the v-bas related sequences to a
3.0-kbp SacI fragment of the T24 oncogene (Santos et al.
1982). Two other laboratories have obtained analogous
results utilizing v-ras as a molecular probe (Der et al.
1982; Parada et al. 1982).

To compare the T24 oncogene with normal human sequences
related to v-bas [designated c-bas(human)], we isolated
c-bas(human) from a library of normal human fetal liver DNA
(Lawn et al. 1978). A recombinant λ Charon 4A phage containing a 19-kbp EcoRI insert of human DNA exhibited a 6.4 kbp
internal BamHI segment that specifically hybridized with
v-bas. This 6.4 kbp BamHI fragment was subsequently subcloned
in pBR322 and a representative plasmid, designated p344,
used for restriction enzyme analysis. As shown in Fig. 5,
the restriction map of this 6.4-kbp BamHI fragment of normal
human DNA closely matched that of the T24 oncogene. In
fact, the only detectable difference between the two molecules
was a 200-bp deletion that mapped between the SphI and ClaI
cleavage sites in c-bas(human) (Fig. 5). Note that this
deletion maps outside the transforming sequences of the T24
oncogene, as well as outside the sequences related to v-bas
(Fig. 5). These results established that c-bas(human) is an
allele of the T24 bladder carcinoma oncogene.

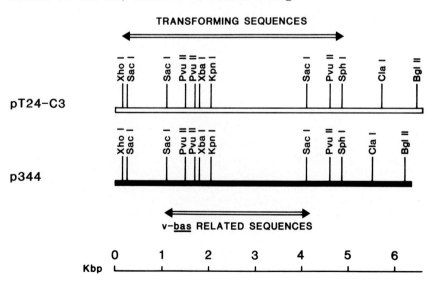

The T24 oncogene has been shown to transform NIH/3T3 cells efficiently, with a specific activity of ~5 x 10^4 focus-forming units/pmol (Goldfarb et al. 1982; Pulciani et al. 1982; Shih, Weinberg 1982). It was of obvious interest to determine whether molecularly cloned c-bas(human) sequences exhibited similar biological activity. As much as 1 µg of c-bas(human) DNA demonstrated no detectable focus-forming activity, whereas in the same experiment, NIH/3T3 cells were readily transformed with as little as 1 ng of the T24 oncogene. The above results, taken together, strongly imply that the acquisition of transforming activity by the T24 oncogene must be the result of subtle genetic alterations (Santos et al. 1982).

Der et al. (1982) have recently reported that oncogenes associated with human lung and colon carcinomas are related to the ras gene of Kirsten-MSV. Similar results have been obtained in our own and at least one other laboratory (Wigler, personal communication). Thus, the homology detected between human oncogenes and retroviral onc genes is not likely to represent a few isolated examples. Whether the battery of available retroviral onc genes will be sufficient to identify all newly identified dominant transforming genes of human tumors remains to be determined. In any case, the distinctions between these two sets of transforming genes appear to be diminishing rapidly. The role of activated or altered human homologues of retroviral onc genes in processes leading to human malignancy obviously requires much further investigation. Nonetheless, it now appears likely that the large fund of knowledge that has been gained from studies of retroviruses over a number of years by many investigators will be directly applicable to studies of naturally occurring tumors of man.

Fig. 5. Comparative restriction maps of the T24 oncogene and c-bas(human). The diagram depicts the location of the cleavage sites for XhoI, SacI, PvuII, XbaI, KpnI, SphI, ClaI and BglII restriction endonucleases within the subcloned BamHI human DNA fragments containing the T24 oncogene (pT24-C3) and c-bas(human) (p344). The location of the transforming sequences of the T24 oncogene and its c-bas (human) related sequence are as indicated.

Aaronson SA, Rowe WP (1970). Nonproducer clones of murine sarcoma virus transformed BALB/3T3 cells. Virology 42:9.

Andersen PR, Devare SG, Tronick SR, Ellis RW, Aaronson SA Scolnick EM (1981). Generation of BALB-MuSV and Ha-MuSV by type C virus transduction of homologous transforming genes from different species. Cell 26:129.

Andersen PR, Tronick SR, Aaronson SA (1981). Structural organization and biological activity of molecular clones of the integrated genome of a BALB/c mouse sarcoma virus (BALB-MSV). J Virol 40:431.

Baltimore D (1974). Tumor viruses. Cold Spring Harbor Symp Quant Biol 39:1187.

Barbacid M, Breitman ML, Lauver AL, Long LK, Vogt PK (1981). The transformation-specific proteins of avian (Fujinami and PRC11) and feline (Snyder-Theilen and Gardner-Arnstein) sarcoma viruses are immunologically related. Virology 110:411.

Beemon K (1981). Transforming proteins of some feline and avian sarcoma viruses are related structurally and functionally. Cell 24:145.

Bernheim A, Berger R, Lenoir G (1981). Cytogenic studies on African Burkitt's lymphoma cell line: t(8;14), t(2;8) and t(8;22) translocation. Cancer Genet and Cytogenet 3:307.

Bishop JM (1978). Retroviruses. Annu Rev Biochem 47:35.

Collet MS, Erickson RL (1978). Protein kinase activity associated with the avian sarcoma virus src gene product. Proc Natl Acad Sci USA 75:2021.

Cooper GM (1982). Cellular transforming genes. Science 218:801.

Dalla-Favera R, Franchini G, Martinotti S, Wong-Staal F, Gallo RC, Croce CM (1982). Chromosomal assignment of the human homologues of feline sarcoma virus and avian myeloblastosis virus onc genes. Proc Natl Acad Sci USA 79:4714.

Der CJ, Krontiris TG, Cooper GM (1982). Transforming genes of human bladder and lung carcinoma cell lines are homologous to the ras genes of Harvey and Kirsten sarcoma viruses. Proc Natl Acad Sci USA 79:3637.

Devare SG, Reddy EP, Robbins KC, Andersen PR, Tronick SR, Aaronson SA (1982). Nucleotide sequence of the transforming gene of simian sarcoma virus. Proc Natl Acad Sci USA 79:3179.

Dhar R, McClements WL, Enquist LW, Vande Woude GW (1980). Nucleotide sequences of integrated Moloney sarcoma provirus long terminal repeats and their host and viral junctions. Proc Natl Acad Sci USA 77:3937.

Dhar R, Ellis R, Shih TY, Oroszlan S, Shapiro B, Maizel J, Lowy D, Scolnick E (1982). Nucleotide sequence of the p21 transforming protein of Harvey murine sarcoma virus. Science 217:934.

Donoghue DJ, Sharp PJ, Weinberg RA (1979). Comparative study of different isolates of murine sarcoma virus. J Virol 32:1015.

Duesberg PH, Vogt PK (1979). Avian acute leukemia viruses MC29 and MH2 share specific RNA sequences: evidence for a second class of tranforming genes. Proc Natl Acad Sci USA 76:1633.

Ellis RW, DeFeo D, Shih TY, Gonda MA, Young HA, Tsuchida N, Lowy DR, Scolnick EM (1981). The p21 src genes of Harvey and Kirsten sarcoma viruses originate from divergent members of a family of normal vertebrate genes. Nature 292:506.

Eva A, Robbins KC, Andersen PR, Srinivasan A, Tronick SR, Reddy EP, Ellmore NW, Galen AT, Lautenberger JA, Papas TS, Westin EH, Wong-Staal F, Gallo RC, Aaronson SA (1982). Cellular genes analogous to retroviral onc genes are transcribed in human tumour cells. Nature 295:116.

Frankel AE, Gilbert JH, Porzig KJ, Scolnick EM, Aaronson SA (1979). Nature and distribution of feline sarcoma virus nucleotide sequences. J Virol 30:821.

Ghysdael J, Neil JC, Vogt PK (1981). A third class of avian sarcoma viruses, defined by related transformation-specific proteins of Yamaguchi 73 and Esh sarcoma viruses. Proc Natl Acad Sci USA 78:2611.

Goldfarb M, Shimizu K, Perucho M, Wigler M (1982). Isolation and preliminary characterization of a human transforming gene from T24 bladder carcinoma cells. Nature 296:404.

Graham FL, van der Eb AJ (1973). Transformation of rat cells by DNA of human adenovirus 5. Virology 52:456.

Hunter T, Sefton BM (1980). The transforming gene product of Rous sarcoma virus phosphorylates tryosine. Proc Natl Acad Sci USA 77:1311.

Kitamura N, Kitamura A, Toyoshima K, Hirayama Y, Yoshida M (1982). Avian sarcoma virus Y73 genome sequence and structural similarity of its transforming gene product to that of Rous sarcoma virus. Nature 297:205.

Klein G (1981). The role of gene dosage and genetic transpositions in carcinogenesis. Nature 294:313.

Lawn RM, Fritsch EF, Parker RC, Blake G, Maniatis T (1978). The isolation and characterization of linked δ- and β-globin genes from a cloned library of human DNA. Cell 15:1157.

Levinson AD, Opperman H, Levintow L, Varmus HE, Bishop JM (1978). Evidence that the transforming gene of avian sarcoma virus encodes a protein kinase associated with a phosphoprotein. Cell 15:561.

Parada LF, Tabin CJ, Shih C, Weinberg RA (1982). Human EJ bladder carcinoma oncogene is homologue of Harvey sarcoma virus ras gene. Nature 297:474.

Prakash K, McBride OW, Swan DC, Devare SG, Tronick SR, Aaronson SA (1982). Molecular cloning and chromosomal mapping of a human locus related to the Moloney murine sarcoma virus transforming gene. Proc Natl Acad Sci USA 79:5210.

Pulciani S, Santos E, Lauver AV, Long LK, Robbins KC, Barbacid M (1982). Oncogenes in human tumor cell lines: molecular cloning of a transforming gene from human bladder carcinoma cells. Proc Natl Acad Sci USA 79:2845.

Rasheed S, Gardner MB, Huebner RJ (1978). In vitro isolation of stable rat sarcoma viruses. Proc Natl Acad Sci USA 75:2972.

Reddy EP, Smith MJ, Aaronson SA (1981). Complete nucleotide sequence and organization of the Moloney murine sarcoma virus genome. Science 214:445.

Robbins KC, Devare SG, Aaronson SA (1981). Molecular cloning of integrated simian sarcoma virus: genome organization of infectious DNA clones. Proc Natl Acad Sci USA 78:2918.

Robbins KC, Devare SG, Reddy EP, Aaronson SA. In vivo identification of the transforming gene product of simian sarcoma virus. Science, in press.

Rowley JD (1980). Chromosome abnormalities in human leukemia. Annu Rev Genet 14:17.

Santos E, Tronick SR, Aaronson SA, Pulciani S, Barbacid M (1982). T24 human bladder carcinoma oncogene is an activated form of the normal human homologue of BALB- and Harvey-MSV transforming genes. Nature 298:343.

Shibuya M, Hanafusa T, Hanafusa H, Stephenson JR (1980). Homology exists among the transforming sequences of avian and feline sarcoma viruses. Proc Natl Acad Sci USA 77:6536.

Shih C, Weinberg RA (1982). Isolation of a transforming sequence from a human bladder carcinoma cell line. Cell 29:161.

Shimotohno K, Mizutani S, Temin HM (1980). Sequence of retro-virus provirus resembles that of bacterial transposable elements. Nature 285:550.

Srinivasan A, Reddy EP, Aaronson SA (1981). Abelson murine leukemia virus: molecular cloning of infectious integrated proviral DNA. Proc Natl Acad Sci USA 78:2077.

Stehelin D, Guntaka RV, Varmus HE, Bishop JM (1976). Purification of DNA complementary to nucleotide sequences required for neoplastic transformation by fibroblasts of avian sarcoma viruses. J Mol Biol 101:349.

Swan DC, McBride OW, Robbins KC, Keithley DA, Reddy EP, Aaronson SA (1982). Chromosomal mapping of the simian sarcoma virus onc gene analogue in human cells. Proc Natl Acad Sci USA 79:4691.

Tronick SR, Robbins KC, Canaani E, Devare S, Andersen PR, Aaronson SA (1979). Molecular cloning of Moloney murine sarcoma virus: arrangement of virus-related sequences within the normal mouse genome. Proc Natl Acad Sci USA 76:6314.

Tsuchida N, Ryder T, Ohtsubo E (1982). Nucleotide sequence of the oncogene encoding the p21 transforming protein of Kirsten murine sarcoma virus. Science 217:937.

Van Beveren C, Galleshaw JA, Jonas V, Berns AJM, Doolittle RF, Donoghue DJ, Verma IM (1981). Nucleotide sequence and formation of the transforming gene of a mouse sarcoma virus. Nature 289:258.

Wang LH (1978). The gene order of avian RNA tumor viruses derived from biochemical analyses of deletion mutants and viral recombinants. Ann Rev Microbiol 32:561.

Westin EH, Wong-Staal F, Gelmann EP, Dalla-Favera R, Papas TS, Lautenberger JA, Eva A, Reddy EP, Tronick SR, Aaronson SA, Gallo RC (1982). Expression of cellular homologues of retroviral onc genes in human hematopoietic cells. Proc Natl Acad Sci USA 79:2490.

Young HA, Rasheed S, Sowder R, Benton CV, Hendersen LE (1981). Rat sarcoma virus: further analysis of individual viral isolates and the gene product. J Virol 38:286.

Young HA, Shih TY, Scolnick EM, Rasheed S, Gardner MB (1979). Different rat-derived transforming retroviruses code for an immunologically related intracellular phosphoprotein. Proc Natl Acad Sci USA 76:3523.

Oncogenes and Retroviruses: Evaluation of Basic Findings
and Clinical Potential, pages 223–242
© 1983 Alan R. Liss, Inc., 150 Fifth Avenue, New York, NY 10011

HUMAN T-CELL LEUKEMIA-LYMPHOMA VIRUS (HTLV) AND HUMAN VIRAL ONC GENE HOMOLOGUES

Robert C. Gallo and Flossie Wong-Staal

Laboratory of Tumor Cell Biology
National Cancer Institute
Bethesda, MD   20205

Retroviruses are etiological agents of naturally occurring leukemias and lymphomas in many animal species (Wong-
Staal and Gallo, in press). Most of these viruses are
"chronic" leukemia viruses. They induce a wide spectrum of
diseases in animals after long latency periods and they do
not transform cells in vitro. These viruses do not contain
genes which code for proteins specific for cellular transformation (onc genes). Another type of leukemia viruses,
known as the "acute" leukemia viruses, has been isolated
from both laboratory induced tumors and, more rarely naturally occurring tumors. The genomes of these viruses contain onc genes which are responsible for rapid tumor induction in vivo and target cell transformation in vitro. All
viral onc genes have been shown to be derived from normal
cellular genes (c-onc genes) of their hosts of origin. Furthermore, all c-onc genes are highly conserved and homologues of each can be identified in all vertebrate species.
Some of these c-onc genes are known to be activated in
tumors induced by the chronic leukemia viruses. For example, avian leukosis virus induced B-cell lymphomas and er-
ythroblastomas express high levels of the onc genes c-myc
and c-erb respectively as a result of provirus integration
near these genes (Hayward et al., 1981; H.J. Kung, personal
communication). It is speculated that in general, chronic
leukemia viruses induce leukemias by activation of cellular
genes which may or may not be homologues of the already
identified viral onc genes. It is conceivable that the target genes for leukemogenic agents (viral or nonviral) could
be those involved in driving proliferation of specific he-

matopoietic cells e.g. growth factor genes. In this paper,
we would like to summarize recent work in our laboratory
dealing with (i) human onc gene homologues, their structure
and expression in human cells, (ii) the characterization of
a human retrovirus associated with mature T-cells and its
possible interaction with the production of or response to
T-cell growth factor (TCGF).

HUMAN C-ONC GENE HOMOLOGUES

    The interest of our laboratory in c-onc genes is chief-
ly in their role in growth, differentiation, and neoplastic
transformation of human cells. We have molecularly cloned
human DNA sequences homologous to sis of simian sarcoma
virus (Dalla-Favera et al., 1981), fes of feline sarcoma
virus (Franchini et al., 1982), myb of avian myeloblastosis
virus (Franchini et al., in preparation), and myc of avian
myelocytomatosis virus MC29 (Dalla Favera et al., in
press a). Studies on the genomic organization of these
genes indicated that they resemble c-onc genes of their
species of origin. As shown in Fig. 1, all four human c-onc
genes contain introns. In the case of c-myc, there is at

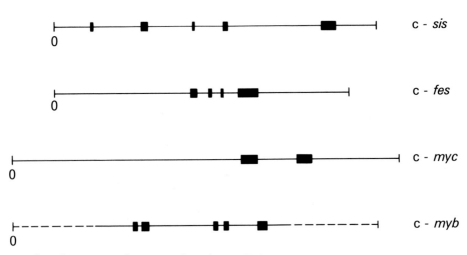

Fig. 1. Genetic organization of four human c-onc loci.
Numbers in parentheses represent the chromosomal location of
the respective c-onc genes. Black boxes denote regions of
homology with the respective v-onc genes.

least one complete human c-myc gene structurally analogous
to chicken c-myc and probably corresponds to the functional
c-myc gene in man. In addition, cloned sequences that are
intronless, divergent and incomplete in their extents of
homology with v-myc have also been obtained, and these most
likely represent amplified myc-related pseudogenes (Dalla
Favera et al., in press a).

The chromosomal locations of myb, fes, sis, and myc
have been assigned to the human chromosomes 6, 15, 22, and 8
respectively (Dalla Favera et al., 1982a; Dalla Favera et
al., in press b and unpublished data). It would be of interest to examine the level of expression and genetic organization of these genes in tumors with specific translocations
involving the specific chromosomes.

EXPRESSION OF ONC GENE HOMOLOGUES IN HUMAN CELLS

We have examined a wide variety of human cells for the
expression of onc genes homologues of Abelson murine leukemia virus (abl), avian myelocytomatosis virus (myc), avian
myeloblastosis virus (myb), Harvey murine sarcoma virus (Ha-
ras), simian sarcoma virus (sis), and feline sarcoma virus
(fes). Molecularly cloned probes containing the v-onc
sequences were labeled and hybridized to poly(A) containing
RNA by the gel blotting technique described by Thomas (1981).

Hematopoietic Cells

Our source of human hematopoietic cells include fresh
uncultured cells from normal individuals and leukemia patients as well as various cell lines of defined marker characteristics representing cells of myeloid, lymphoid and erythroid lineages arrested at different stages of differentiation. The results (Westin et al., 1982a, 1982b) are summarized in Table 1. Several points can be generalized from
these studies: (1) There is no obvious difference between
fresh and cultured cells of the same lineage, e.g., fresh
AML cells and T-ALL cells behave as myeloblast cell lines
(KG-1) and T-lymphoblast lines (CCRF-CEM, Molt-4) respectively. This argues for the validity of studying cell lines
in these experiments. (2) The size(s) of mRNA for a given
onc gene is the same in all human cells, and very similar

(though not necessarily identical) to that of mRNA in other vertebrate cells. (3) The patterns of expression of different onc genes vary. Thus, each c-onc gene should be considered separate from the others. Specifically, the abl and Ha-ras genes are detectably expressed (1-5 copies per cell) in all hematopoietic cells examined as multiple mRNA species. These genes are probably important for some basic cellular functions. The myc and myb genes code for single size transcripts of 2.7 Kb and 4.5 Kb respectively. However, the expression of myb is more restricted than myc. The myc gene is transcribed in all hematopoietic cells examined, including normal peripheral blood lymphocytes prior to or after stimulation with PHA. The only exception is terminally differentiated HL60 cells where myc transcription is turned off. The myb gene is expressed in the early precursor cells of lymphoid, myeloid, and erythroid lineages, but there is little or no expression relatively early in B-lymphoid cells differentiation, and late in T-cell or myeloid cell differentiation. Like myc, myb is transcribed in undifferentiated HL60 cells but not in HL60 cells induced to differentiate with either DMSO or retinoic acid. The sis and fes genes are not commonly transcribed in hematopoietic cells. There are two instances where enhanced transcription is observed: myc transcription in the promyelocytic cell line HL60 and myb transcription in leukemic T-lymphoblasts. However, it is premature to conclude that these enhanced expressions are disease related. Normal cells of equivalent lineages and stages of differentiation and/or more samples of similar disease types will be needed to further clarify the correlation.

Solid Tumors

A parallel study of human solid tumors and normal fibroblast cell lines has been carried out in collaboration with others and in particular S. Aaronson and colleagues (Eva et al., 1981). The results reinforced the universality of expression of abl and Ha-ras genes. The myb gene is not expressed in these cells and may be specifically involved in hematopoietic cell differentiation. Of interest is the finding that c-sis is frequently expressed at moderate to high levels in sarcomas and glioblastomas but not in any melanomas, carcinomas or normal fibroblast cell lines. Therefore, expression of this gene shows the greatest correlation with specific types of neoplasias.

TABLE 1

EXPRESSION OF onc GENES IN HUMAN HEMATOPOIETIC CELLS*

Cell Type	Source	Stage of Differentiation	mRNA Species Detected with					
			v-abl (Kb) 7.2, 6.4 3.8 & 2.0	v-myc (Kb) 2.7	v-myb (Kb) 4.5	v-Ha-ras (Kb) 6.5 5.8 & 1.5	v-sis (Kb) 4.3	v-fes ?
Myeloid	KG-1, Fresh AML	Myeloblast	++	++	++	+	−	−
	HL60	Promyelocyte	++	++++	++	+	−	−
	HL60 + DMSO, RA	Granulocyte	++	+/−	−	+	−	−
Erythroid	K562	(Immature Erythroid Precursor)	++	++	++	+	−	−
Lymphoid T-cells:	CEM, MOLT 4 FRESH ALL	Immature T-Cell	++	++	+++	+	−	−
	HUT78	Mature T-cell	++	++	−	+	−	−
	HUT102	Mature T-cell	++	++	−	+	+	−
B-cells:	Raji, Daudi	Burkitt Lymphoma	++	++	−	+	−	−
	NC37, CRB	EBV Transformed	++	++	−	+	−	−
	Normal Peripheral Lymphocytes		NT	++	−	NT	NT	NT
	Normal Peripheral Lymphocytes + PHA		NT	++	−	NT	NT	NT

NT = Not Tested.

* Taken from Westin et al. (1982a, 1982b).

C-MYC AMPLIFICATION IN HL60

    To investigate whether any structural alterations of
the c-myc gene could account for increased levels of c-myc
expression in HL60, we analyzed HL60 DNA by Southern blot
hybridization to v-myc (Dalla Favera et al., 1982b). The
probe used detected all c-myc related sequences in the human
genome, including the pseudogenes. As shown in Fig. 2, a
12.8 Kb EcoRI band corresponding to the complete, presumably
functional gene was markedly increased in DNA from both primary and cultured HL60 cells as compared to DNA from other
normal or leukemic individuals. In contrast, the intensity

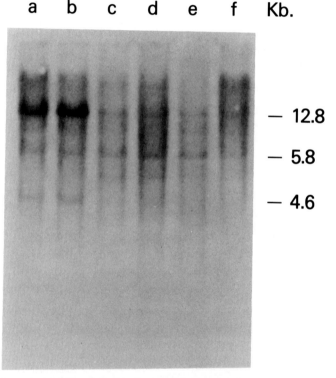

Fig. 2. Amplification of c-myc in HL60.
Thirty µg of DNA from a) HL60 passage 70; b) primary HL-60
leukemic cells; c) normal human spleen; d) peripheral blood
AML cells; e) an immature T-cell lines, Molt 4; f) peripheral blood normal human lymphocytes were digested with
EcoRI and hybridized to a v-myc probe (pMCo) (Dalla-Favera
et al., 1982b).

of a 5.8 Kb band, which corresponds to one of the c-myc pseudogenes, is uniform in all the samples. This result suggests that only the functional gene, but not the pseudogenes, is amplified.

Experiments to quantitate the amplification of c-myc in HL60 indicate that the c-myc gene is amplified between 16 and 32-fold. The levels of c-myc amplification do not seem to vary during prolonged cell culture or after induction to differentiation when the c-myc gene is no longer expressed. The amplification of c-myc cannot be simply explained by amplification of specific chromosome(s) in these cells since they are hypodiploid and no hyperdiploidy of individual chromosomes was present (Gallagher et al., 1979). Since tissues other than the leukemic cells are not available from the patient we cannot determine whether c-myc was amplified in the other nonleukemic cells of the same individual. There is no definitive proof that amplification of c-myc is causally linked to the disease in the patient HL60. However, the genetic modification of a known onc gene resulting in high level expression of this gene which can be turned off when the cells are induced to differentiate into phenotypically "normal" cells argued for a role of c-myc in the patient's disease. On the other hand, recent data from Weinberg's group (see Dautry et al., this symposium) showed that the gene in HL60 that transforms mouse NIH3T3 cells in vitro is not c-myc. This raises the question which or if either of these two genes is the relevant "transforming" gene in the primary disease.

PROLIFERATION OF NORMAL AND LEUKEMIC MATURE T-LYMPHOCYTES: THE ROLE OF TCGF

We will now focus on one particular hematopoietic cell system, the mature T-lymphocyte. The proliferation of mature T-cells normally involves at least three major steps (Ruscetti and Gallo, 1981): (1) activation of a subset of T-cells by an antigen or lectin to synthesize receptor for TCGF; (2) interaction of an antigent or lectin with an adherent cell and a different subset of T-cells to produce TCGF; and (3) interaction of the activated (receptor-positive) T-cells with TCGF leading to T-cell proliferation. Subsequent to the discovery of TCGF, partially purified TCGF has been used to expand normal T-cells in vitro. It was also observed that some neoplastic mature T-cells possess TCGF receptors without prior lectin or antigen activation. A number of neoplastic T-cell lines have been established by direct exposure to TCGF (Gazdar et al., 1980; Poiesz et al., 1980a; Popovic et al., submitted). These cells are generally pleomorphic with convoluted nuclei. Once established in culture, they exhibited a decline in dependence for exogenous TCGF. A few became entirely independent of TCGF. So far, cell lines have been established from patients with a variety of mature T-cell malignancies diagnosed as cutaneous T-cell lymphoma, Sézary leukemia, adult T-cell leukemia, peripheral T-cell lymphoma, etc. There are many common clinical features associated with these diseases which may represent a specific subtype of mature T-cell malignancy. In almost all cases, the established cell lines were found to be positive for a novel retrovirus that we named human T-cell leukemia-lymphoma virus (HTLV) (Poiesz et al., 1980b; Poiesz et al., 1981; Popovic et al., submitted).

DIFFERENT ISOLATES OF HTLV

Subsequent to the initial isolation of HTLV from a US black patient with CTCL in 1978 (Poiesz et al., 1980b) and the extensive characterization that HTLV is distinct from all known animal retroviruses (Reitz et al., 198]; Kalyanaraman et al., 1981a; Rho et al., 1981), many additional isolates have been obtained from patients all over the world (Poiesz et al., 1981; Hinuma et al., 1981; Gallo et al., 1982; Yoshida et al., 1982; Popovic et al., submitted) (Table 2). All cell lines have karyotype and HLA patterns that match those of the donors, and the HLA profiles are different for all cell lines. These patients include four individuals from the United States, one from Israel and three from a single Japanese family from the northwest part of the Thousand Islands in Japan. In this family, the patient SK has acute T-cell lymphoma (ATL) and both his parents and a brother are virus positive. The father (MK) is clinically healthy and the mother (TK) has persistent lymphocytosis, which is considered to be a preleukemic state (Aoki et al., in press). In addition, a T-cell line established by Golde and colleagues from a patient (MO) with hairy cell leukemia (Saxon et al., 1978) was positive for HTLV p19 and p24 (Kalyanaraman et al., 1982a). We propose to designate each virus isolate with a subscript of the

TABLE 2

Expression of new HTLV isolates in T-cell lines
derived from patients with adult T-cell leukemia/lymphomas

Cell Line[4]	p24[1] (ng/mg)	p19 (% Positive Cells)	RT Activity[3] (pmoles/ml extract)	EM
MJ	128	85	9.3	+
UK	1941	71	4.5	+
MI	1503	63	16.8	+
WA	1076	78	19.2	+
PL	683	23	6.2	+
SK	174	39	5.8	+
TK	2700	54	33.0	+
HK	400	38	13.5	+

[1]Detected by competitive radioimmunoprecipitation assay
(RIPA) in cell extract.
[2]Indirect immunofluoresence assay (IFA).
[3]Reverse transcriptase activity (RTA) in culture fluids was
measured with $(dt)^{15} (rA)_n$.
[4]Cell lines were derived from peripheral blood (PB) or bone
marrow (BM) of different patients as follows: (a) MJ from PB
of a 50 yr old white male with mycosis fungoides, from Boston, Massachusetts; (b) UK from PB of a 45 yr old white male
with diffuse histiocytic lymphoma, from Jerusalem, Israel;
(c) MI from PB of a 32 yr old black female with T-cell lym-
phosarcoma cell leukemia, from Granada, West Indies; (d) WA
from BM of a 24 yr old black male with diffuse mixed lymphoma, from Augusta, Georgia;(e) PL from PB of a 27 yr old
black female with T-cell diffuse mixed lymphoma. from Ovita,
Florida; (f) SK from PB of a 21 yr old male with adult T-
cell leukemia, from Akita prefecture, Japan; (g) TK from PB
of a 45 yr old female (mother of patient SK) who has 7% abnormal cells in her blood, from Akita prefecture, Japan; and
(h) HK from PB of a 49 yr old male (father of patient SK)
who is normal, from Akita prefecture, Japan.

patient's initials, e.g., $HTLV_{CR}$, $HTLV_{MB}$, etc. All isolates except $HTLV_{MO}$ are highly related to each other as assayed by competitive radioimmunoassay with p24 and hybridization of viral cDNA to mRNA of the producer cell lines (Reitz et al., in preparation). By these assays, the virus of Japanese ATL is indistinguishable from the prototype HTLV as exemplified by the earlier isolates $HTLV_{CR}$ and $HTLV_{MB}$. On the other hand, $HTLV_{MO}$ competes poorly in the p24 assay and nucleic acid sequence homology with $HTLV_{CR}$ was detected only under very non-stringent hybridization conditions (our unpublished data). Therefore, this virus may form a distinct subgroup in the HTLV family. We propose to group them as $HTLV-I_{CR}$, $HTLV-I_{MB}$, etc. versus $HTLV-II_{MO}$.

HTLV PROVIRUS IN NEOPLASTIC T-CELLS: EVIDENCE FOR EXOGENOUS INFECTION AND MONOCLONALITY OF THE INFECTED CELLS

We had reported earlier that HTLV sequences are present in the infected cells and not in normal uninfected human cells (Reitz et al., 1981), suggesting that HTLV is not an endogenous human virus. In the case of the patient CR, we also had the opportunity to find out whether he was infected pre-or post zygotically (Gallo et al., 1982). Several T-cell lines, some clonal derivatives of these lines and a B-cell line have been established from CR. These cells were shown to have originated from the same individual by HLA-typing. HTLV proviral DNA was detected in some but not all of the independently established T-cell lines of CR and not in the B-cells. Furthermore, the surface phenotype OKT3-, OKT4+ and OKT8- appears to correlate with the presence of HTLV. These results indicate that HTLV was acquired by CR by horizontal transmission and suggest that only a subtype of T-cells is the target for HTLV infection.

Recently, molecularly cloned sequences representing the 5' and 3' ends of HTLV have been obtained in our laboratory (V. Manzari et al., submitted). These clones have been used as probes for Southern hybridization of fresh leukemic DNA from patients with HTLV positive diseases (Wong-Staal et al., submitted). These revealed one or few copies of HTLV integrated at a site which is unique for a given patient but varies from patient to patient (Fig. 3). DNA from normal people did not contain hybridizing sequences. A similar observation has been made by others (Yoshida et al., 1982).

These results suggest that the infected cells are of clonal origin, so infection must have occurred prior to disease development. This feature is also found in animal leukemias-lymphomas induced by chronic leukemia retrovirus.

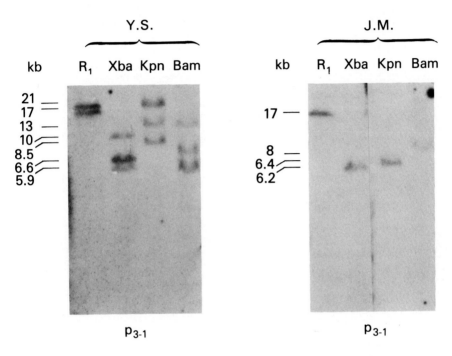

Fig. 3. Detection of HTLV-related sequences in two Japanese ATL patients.

DNA from leukemia cells of two ATL patients was digested with the enzymes as indicated and hybridized to a cloned HTLV probe. (Wong-Staal et al., submitted).

SPECIFIC ANTIBODIES TO HTLV IN HUMAN SERA

Because of the exogenous nature of HTLV, one of the most rapid means to survey for virus infection is to assay sera samples for specific antibodies to HTLV antigens. Five different assays were set up for this seroepidemiologic survey, the most relied on assay being radioimmunoprecipitation using homogeneously purified iodinated core antigen p24. These tests have uncovered different pockets of HTLV infection throughout the world (Posner et al., 1981; Kalyanaraman et al., 1981b; Hinuma et al., 1981; Robert-Guroff et al., 1982; Kalyanaraman et al., 1982b; Catovsky et al., 1982; Blattner et al., 1982; Gallo et al., in press). Table 3 summarizes the findings compiled up to a few months ago. Although the numbers of samples tested have increased by this time, the percentage of positive samples in each category still holds. Two groups stand out in their tight association with HTLV: The Caribbean T-LCL patients and the Japanese ATL patients. Healthy relatives of HTLV-positive patients have a greater than usual chance of having antibodies against HTLV. In areas where the HTLV-associated disease is endemic, a significant number of random healthy donors also have circulating antibodies against HTLV.

TABLE 3

Prevalence of Natural Antibodies to HTLV in Sera of Patients with Malignancies of Mature T-cells, their Healthy Relatives, and Random Normal Donors

| Serum Donors | Antibodies to HTLVα | |
	#Positive/#Tested	% Positive
Healthy Relatives of US Patients with HTLV-associated malignancy	2/12	17
Unrelated Healthy Donors, Washington, D.C.	1/185	<1
Unrelated Healthy Donors, Georgia	3/158	2
Caribbean T-LCL Patients	8/8	100
Healthy Relatives of Caribbean Patients	3/16	19
Random Healthy Donors, Caribbean	12/337	4
Japanese ATL Patients	40/46	87
Healthy Relatives of ATL Patients	19/40	48
Random Healthy Donors, non-endemic area	9/600	2
Random Healthy Donors, endemic area	62/499	12

αAntibodies were detected by RIP of HTLV p24 or by the solid-phase RIA.

INFECTION AND TRANSFORMATION OF HUMAN CORD BLOOD T-CELLS BY
HTLV <u>IN</u> <u>VITRO</u>

Seven of the HTLV isolates described above have been
successfully transmitted into fresh human cord blood T-cells
by cocultivation (Popovic <u>et</u> <u>al</u>., submitted). The virus
positive neoplastic cells used as donors were first treated
with mitomycin-C or X-irradiation before cocultivation with
recipient cord blood cells. After four weeks, assays for T-
cell markers, HTLV, karyotype and HLA-typing were performed.
As shown in Table 4, all recipient cord blood are mature T-
cells, positive for HTLV provirus, and express various
levels of HTLV antigens (p19, p24 and RT). Karyotype and
HLA typing consistently matched the recipient cells. Since
cord blood T-cells from the same donors were consistently
negative for HTLV markers and the plasma from their cord
blood were also negative for HTLV antibodies, we conclude
that the virus was transmitted from HTLV producing neoplastic T-cell lines into cord blood recipient T-cells.
Transmission of HTLV to normal cord blood T-cells was also
reported by Miyoshi <u>et</u> <u>al</u>., 1982

To characterize further whether a target for HTLV could
represent a certain subset of mature T-cells, phenotype of
HTLV producing cells were analyzed by a series of monoclonal
antibodies specific for helper/inducer and suppressor/cyto-
toxic T-cells. We found that a majority of HTLV producing
T-cell lines consistently exhibited only helper-inducer phenotype. Two established T-cell lines SK and TK, both from
Japanese patients and two HTLV infected cord blood T-cells
(C1 and C5) revealed "double" phenotype. However, none of
the T-cell lines exhibited pure suppressor/cytotoxic phenotype. Unlike HTLV infected cord blood T-cells, PHA stimulated cells (control) consist of 70% helper/inducer and 30% of
T-cells with suppressor/cytotoxic phenotype. Thus, these
data from T-cell phenotype characterization of HTLV infected
T-cells again suggest that a certain subset of mature T-
cells is the target for HTLV. HTLV infection studies with
cord blood cells deprived of T-cell population with helper/
inducer of suppressor/cytotoxic phenotype are currently
being carried out.

HTLV-infected cord blood T-cells differ from mitogen
stimulated cord blood T-cells in several growth properties
and cell surface characteristics, the infected cells resem-

bling more the neoplastic cells transformed in vivo by HTLV
(Popovic et al., in preparation). The most striking feature
of HTLV infected cord blood T-cells is their potential for
indefinite growth as shown in Fig. 4. In contrast, mitogen
stimulated cord blood T-cells from the same patients consistently exhibited growth "crises" after one month in culture,
even in the continued presence of TCGF. Furthermore, the
infected cells, like the neoplastic cells, had the tendency
to form clumps in culture. When analyzed by electron microscopy, the cells were seen to have convoluted nuclei (not
shown) while the mitogen stimulated cells were not. Another
important and reproducible difference is the decrease in
requirement for TCGF by the infected cells. In fact, some
of the infected cells are completely independent of exogenous TCGF. Other changes of the infected cells include al-

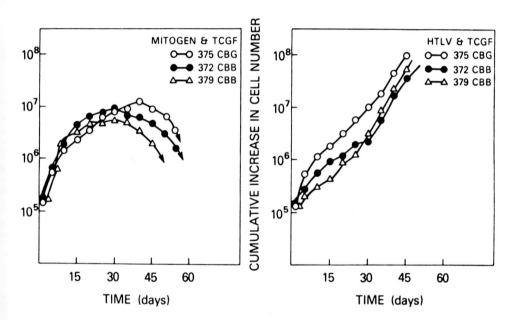

Fig. 4. Growth curves of uninfected and HTLV infected cord
blood T-cells.
    Left panel: Mitogen stimulated cord blood T-cells.
    Right panel: HTLV infected cord blood T-cells.
    C6/WA and C7/TK cell lines are primary cocultures (for
details see Table 4). C5/MJ cells were obtained in three
successive transmissions of HTLV$_{MJ}$ into cord blood cells.

TABLE 4

Transmission of HTLV into human cord blood T-cells

Co-cultured Cells (Recipient X Donor)*	Infected Cells	Karyotype After Co-cultivation**	HTLV Proteins	Expression of HTLV Proteins			
				p19 (%Positive Cells)	p24 (ng/mg)	RTA (pm/ml extract)	EM
C1(F) X None			-	0	<1		
C1(F) X MJ(M)	C1/MJ	XX	+	90	385	3.3	+
C4(F) X None			-	0	<1		
C4(F) X UK(M)	C4/UK	XX	+	81	540	34.1	+
C21(M) X None			-	0	<1		
C21(M) X MI(F)	C21/MK	XY	+	47	235	60.4	+
C6(F) X None			-	0	<1		
C6(F) X WA(M)	C6/WA	XX	+	53	502	1.7	+
C8(F) X None			-	0	<1		
C8(F) X SK(M)	C8/SK	XX	+	47	1000	8.7	+
C7(M) X None			-	0	<1		
C7(M) X TK(F)	C7/TK	XY	+	75	685	84.2	+
C36(F) X None			-	0	ND		
C36(F) X MO(M)	C36/MO	XX		47	500	30.3	ND

*Mitomycin treated or X-ray irradiated.

** 50 to 100 mitoses were analyzed.

(F) = Female

(M) = Male

ND = Not done

teration in their HLA profile and expression of receptors for transferrin, TCGF and HAA (human activated lymphocyte antigen detected by monoclonal antibodies) in a high percentage of cells. The data indicate that HTLV is capable of causing morphological transformation of cord blood T-cells in vitro.

POSSIBLE MOLECULAR MECHANISM OF TRANSFORMATION BY HTLV

As mentioned earlier, analysis of HTLV-positive leukemic T-cells showed that the cells are of clonal origin with respect to the provirus integration sites. In animal systems monoclonality has also been shown to be a common feature of leukemias induced by retroviruses which are chronic leukemia viruses but not those induced by retroviruses which are acute leukemia viruses. Consequently, in spite of its high efficiency to transform T-cells in vitro, HTLV probably does not carry an onc gene. Several chronic leukemia viruses are known to induce leukemia by activating cellular onc genes (myc in B-cell lymphomas and erb in erythroleukemias) (Hayward et al., 1981; Kung personal communication) by integrating in the proximity of these genes. Activation of these genes is brought about by providing either a viral promoter or viral "enhancer" nucleotide sequences (Payne et al., 1982; Levinson et al., 1982). Since HTLV specifically transforms mature T-cells, it is likely to affect expression of genes that are important in T-cell proliferation. A model has been proposed for the mechanism of leukemogenesis by HTLV (Gallo and Wong-Staal, 1982) in which the HTLV provirus integrates in the vicinity of a gene important in T-cell proliferation (e.g. TCGF, TCGF receptor or a gene that exerts a pleitropic effect on TCGF expression or response) and activates that gene by direct promotion or enhancement. The end result is a cell producing both TCGF and TCGF receptor, leading to autostimulation and increased cell proliferation. As an approach to study the gene(s) activated by HTLV infection, we have recently identified and isolated a gene that is expressed at high levels in all HTLV positive neoplastic T-cells and in normal cord blood T-cells after infection with HTLV but not the uninfected counterparts (Manzari et al., in press). Study of the expression pattern of this gene in uninfected human hematopoietic cells suggests that its expression may be linked to TCGF production. Experiments are in progress to determine if HTLV integrates at a preferred locus in the human chromosome and affects transcription of specific cellular genes in the vicinity, including this gene in question.

Acknowledgments

We would like to acknowledge our colleagues for contributing to the data presented here, especially R. Dalla Favera, M. Popovic, V. Manzari, and G. Franchini for permission to quote their unpublished data. We also thank Jessie Blalock and Vicki Sutton for preparation of the manuscript.

Aoki T, Shibata H, Ohnishi Y, Aoyagi Y, Miyakoshi H, Emura I, Kalyanaraman VS, Robert-Guroff M, Popovic M, Sarngadharan M, Sarin PS, Nowell PC, Gallo RC. High incidence of the Human Type-C retrovirus (HTLV) in Family members of an HTLV-positive Japanese T-cell leukemia patient and indications of a preleukemic state in one member. Proc Nat Acad Sci USA (in press).

Catovsky D, Greaves MF, Rose M, Galton DAG, Goolden AWG, McCluskey DR, White JM, Lampert I, Bourikas G, Ireland R, Brownell AI, Bridges JM, Blattner WA, Gallo RC (1982). Adult T-cell lymphoma-leukemia in blacks from the West Indies. Lancet I (#8273):639-642.

Dalla Favera R, Gelmann EP, Gallo RC, Wong-Staal F (1981). A human onc gene homologous to the transforming gene (v-sis) of simian sarcoma virus. Nature 292:31-35.

Dalla Favera R, Franchini G, Martinotti S, Wong-Staal F, Gallo R, Croce CM (1982a). Chromosomal assignment of the human homologues of feline sarcoma virus and avian myeloblastosis virus onc genes. Proc Natl Acad Sci USA 79:4714-4717.

Dalla Favera R, Wong-Staal F, Gallo RC (1982b). Onc gene amplification in promyelocytic leukaemia cell line HL-60 and primary leukaemic cells of the same patient. Nature 299:61-63.

Dalla Favera R, Gelmann EP, Martinotti S, Franchini G, Papas TS, Gallo RC, Wong-Staal F (1982). Cloning and characterization of different human sequences related to the onc-gene (v-myc) of avian myelocytomatosis virus (MC29). Proc Natl Acad Sci USA (in press a).

Dalla Favera R, Gallo RC, Giallongo A, Croce CM (1982). Chromosomal localization of the human homologue (c-sis) of the simian sarcoma virus onc-gene. Science (in press b).

Eva A, Robbins KC, Andersen PR, Srinvasan A, Tronick SR, Ready EP, Ellmore NW, Galen AT, Lautenberger JA, Papas TS, Westin EH, Wong-Staal F, Gallo RC, Aaronson SA (1981). Cellular genes analogous to retroviral onc genes are transcribed in human tumor cells. Nature 95:116-119.

Franchini G, Gelmann EP, Dalla Favera R, Gallo RC, Wong-Staal F (1982). A human gene (c-fes) related to the onc sequences of Snyder-Theilen feline sarcoma virus. Mol Cell Biol 2:1014-1019.

Gallagher R, Collins S, Trujillo J, McCredie K, Ahearn M, Tsai S, Metzgar R, Aulakh G, Ting R, Ruscetti F, Gallo RC (1979). Characterization of the continuous differentiating myeloid cell line (HL-60) from a patient with acute promyelocytic leukemia. Blood 54:713-733.

Gallo RC, Wong-Staal F (1982). Retroviruses as etiologic agents of some animal and human leukemias and lymphomas and as tools for elucidating the molecular mechanism of leukemogenesis. Blood 60:545-557.

Gallo RC, Mann D, Broder S, Ruscetti FW, Maeda M, Kalyanaraman VS, Robert-Guroff M, Reitz MS, Jr. (1982). Human T-cell leukemia-lymphoma virus (HTLV) is in T but not B-lymphocytes from a patient with cutaneous T-cell lymphoma. Proc Natl Acad Sci USA 79:5680-5683.

Gallo RC et al. (1982). The human type-C retrovirus: association with a subset of adult T-cell malignancies. N Engl J Med (in press).

Gazdar AF, Carney DN, Bunn PA, Russell EK, Jaffe ES, Schechter GP, Guccion JG (1980). Blood 55:409-417.

Hayward WS, Neel BG, Astrin SM (1981). Induction of lymphoid leukosis by avian leukosis virus: activation of a cellular "onc" gene by promoter insertion. Nature 290: 475-480.

Hinuma Y, Nagata K, Hanaoka M, Nakai M, Matsumoto T, Kinoshita K, Shirakawa S, Miyoshi I (1981). Adult T-cell leukemia: antigen in an ATL cell line and detection of antibodies to the antigen in human sera. Proc Nat Acad Sci USA 78:6476-6480.

Kalyanaraman VS, Sarngadharan MG, Poiesz BJ, Ruscetti FW, Gallo RC (1981a). Immunological properties of a type-C retrovirus isolated from cultured human T-lymphoma cells and comparison to other mammalian retroviruses. J Virol 38:906-913.

Kalyanaraman VS, Sarngadharan MG, Bunn PA, Minna JD, Gallo RC (1981b). Antibodies in human sera reactive against an internal structural protein of human T-cell lymphoma virus. Nature 294:271-273.

Kalyanaraman VS, Sarngadharan MG, Robert-Guroff M, Miyoshi I, Blayney D, Golde D, Gallo RC (1982a). A new subtype of human T-cell leukemia-lymphoma virus (HTLV-II) associated with a T-cell variant of Hairy cell leukemia. Science (in press).

Kalyanaraman VS, Sarngadharan MG, Nakao Y, Ito Y, Aoki T, Gallo RC (1982b). Natural antibodies to the structural core protein (p24) of the human T-cell leukemia (lymphoma) retrovirus (HTLV) found in sera of leukemic patients in Japan. Proc Natl Acad Sci USA 79:1653-1657.

Levinson B, Khoury G, Vande Woude G, Gruss P (1982). Activation of SV40 genome by 72 base pair tandem repeats by Moloney sarcoma virus. Nature 295:568-572.

Manzari V, Gallo RC, Franchini G, Westin E, Ceccherini-Nelli L, Popovic M, Wong-Staal F (1982). Abundant transcription of a cellular gene in T-cells infected with human T-cell leukemia-lymphoma virus (HTLV). Proc Natl Acad Sci, in press.

Miyoshi I, Kubonishi I, Yoshimoto S, Akagi T, Ohtsuki Y, Shiraishi Y, Nagata K, Hinuma Y (1981). Type C virus particles in a cord T-cell line derived by co-cultivating normal human cord leukocytes and human leukemic T-cells. Nature 294:770-771.

Payne GS, Courtneidge SA, Crittenden LB, Fedly AM, Bishop JM, Varmus HE (1981). Analysis of avian leukosis virus DNA and RNA in bursal tumors: viral gene expression is not required for maintenance of the tumor state. Cell 23:311-322.

Poiesz BJ, Ruscetti FW, Mier JW, Woods AM, Gallo RC (1980a). T-cell lines established from human T-lymphocytic neoplasias by direct response to T-cell growth factor. Proc Natl Acad Sci USA 77:6815-6819.

Poiesz BJ, Ruscetti FW, Gazdar AF, Bunn PA, Minna JD, Gallo RC (1980b). Isolation of type-C retrovirus particles from cultured and fresh lymphocytes of a patient with cutaneous T-cell lymphoma. Proc Natl Acad Sci USA 77:7415-7419.

Poiesz BJ, Ruscetti FW, Reitz MS, Kalyanaraman VS, Gallo RC (1981). Isolation of a new type-C retrovirus (HTLV) in primary uncultured cells of a patient with Sézary T-cell leukaemia. Nature 294:268-271.

Posner LE, Robert-Guroff M, Kalyanaraman VS, Poiesz BJ, Ruscetti FW, Fossieck B, Bunn PA, Minna JD, Gallo RC (1981). Natural antibodies to the human T-cell lymphoma virus in patients with cutaneous T-cell lymphomas. J Exp Med 154:333-346.

Reitz MS, Poiesz BJ, Ruscetti FW, Gallo RC (1981). Characterization and distribution of nucleic acid sequences of a
novel type-C retrovirus isolated from neoplastic human T-
lymphocytes. Proc Natl Acad Sci USA 78:1887-1891.
Rho HM, Poiesz BJ, Ruscetti FW, Gallo RC (1981). Characterization of the reverse transcriptase from a new retrovirus
(HTLV) produced by a human cutaneous T-cell lymphoma cell
line. Virology 112:355-358.
Robert-Guroff M, Nakao Y, Notake K, Ito Y, Sliski A, Gallo
RC (1982). Natural antibodies to human retrovirus HTLV in
a cluster of Japanese patients with adult T-cell leukemia.
Science 215:975-978.
Ruscetti FW, Gallo RC (1981). Human T-lymphocyte growth
factor: the second signal in the immune response. Blood
57:379-393.
Saxon A, Stevens RH, Golde DW (1978). T-lymphocyte variant
of Hairy cell leukemia. Ann Int Med 88:323-326.
Thomas PS (1980). Hybridization of denatured RNA and small
DNA fragments transformed to nitrocellulose. Proc Natl
Acad Sci USA 77:5201-5205.
Westin EH, Gallo RC, Arya SK, Eva A, Souza LM, Baluda MA,
Aaronson SA, Wong-Staal F (1982b). Differential expres-
sion of the amv gene in human hematopoietic cells. Proc
Natl Acad Sci USA 79:2194-2198.
Westin EH, Wong-Staal F, Gelmann EP, Dalla Favera R, Papas
TS, Lautenberger JA, Eva A, Reddy P, Tronick SR, Aaronson
SA, Gallo RC (1982). Expression of cellular homologues of
retroviral onc genes in human hematopoietic cells. Proc
Natl Acad Sci USA 79:2490-2494.
Wong-Staal F, Gallo RC (1982). Retroviruses and leukemia.
In Gunz F, Henderson E (eds.) "Leukemia", Grune and Strat-
ton, New York (in press).
Wong-Staal F, Hahn B, Manzari V, Colombini S, Franchini G,
Gelmann EP, Gallo RC. A molecular epidemiological survey
of human leukemic cells using cloned DNA sequences of a
human retrovirus, HTLV. Submitted.
Yoshida M, Miyoshi I, Hinuma Y (1982). Isolation and char-
acterization of retrovirus from cell lines of human adult
T-cell leukemia and its implication in the disease. Proc
Natl Acad Sci USA 79:2031-2035.

**Oncogenes and Retroviruses: Evaluation of Basic Findings
and Clinical Potential, pages 243–249**
© **1983 Alan R. Liss, Inc., 150 Fifth Avenue, New York, NY 10011**

ISOLATION OF ATLV FROM HEALTHY ATLV CARRIERS BY MIXED LYM-
PHOCYTE CULTURE

Isao Miyoshi, M.D., Hirokuni Taguchi, M.D.,
Yuji Ohtsuki, M.D. and Yukimasa Shiraishi, Ph.D.

Kochi Medical School
Kochi 781-51, Japan

Adult T-cell leukemia (ATL) virus (ATLV) was detected
in short-term or long-term cultures of leukemic cells from
patients with ATL (Akagi et al 1982; Hinuma et al 1981;
Hinuma et al 1982). A similar virus, HTLV, was independently isolated from patients with cutaneous T-cell lymphoma
(Poiesz et al 1980; Poiesz et al 1981). Co-cultivation of
ATL cells and human cord blood leukocytes led to the establishment of an ATLV-carrying cord T-cell line (Miyoshi et al
1981a). All these cultures contained ATL-associated antigens (ATLA)-positive cells which reacted specifically with
sera from ATL patients. Recently, we have detected ATLV in
phytohemagglutinin-stimulated short-term cultures of peripheral lymphocytes from anti-ATLA positive healthy individuals
(Miyoshi et al 1982a; Miyoshi et al 1982b). This paper reports isolation of ATLV-producing T-cell lines by mixed lymphocyte culture between anti-ATLA positive and negative
healthy adults.

Blood was collected from three anti-ATLA positive fe-
males and two anti-ATLA negative males. The female donors
are sisters (B and D) and wife (E) of an ATL patient and
were shown to be the healthy carriers of ATLV (Miyoshi et al
1982b). The male donors (TK and MF) who are both collaborators of this work are also healthy. Mononuclear leukocytes were separated from 10 ml of peripheral blood by
Ficoll-Hypaque gradient centrifugation. The leukocytes from
anti-ATLA positive donors were cultured at 1×10^6/ml in 35-
mm Petri dishes with RPMI 1640 medium supplemented with 10%
human cord serum, 10% fetal calf serum, and antibiotics.
After 3-7 days, leukocytes from anti-ATLA negative donors

were added at 1 x 10^6/ml to the dishes. The leukocytes from
both anti-ATLA positive and negative donors were also cultured alone at 1 x 10^6/ml as controls. All cultures were
incubated at 37°C in a humidified 7.5% atmosphere and partial medium changes were done twice a week.

One to two weeks after co-culture, clumps of cells were
formed and gradually increased in size and number. The
cells were first subcultured 2-4 weeks after co-culture and
have since been maintained in continuous culture for over
eight months. The three cell lines thus established by
mixed lymphocyte culture were designated Ha, As and Ei.
These cell lines grew in suspension forming clumps of cells
and consisted of mostly immature lymphoid cells. The leukocytes from all donors cultured alone degenerated by two
months.

Ha, As and Ei cells formed spontaneous rosettes with
neuraminidase-treated sheep erythrocytes and reacted with
monoclonal antibodies to T-cells (Leu-1) and Ia antigens
(OKI1). They were all negative for Epstein-Barr virus nuclear antigen. Chromosome analysis of Ha and As showed
normal female karyotypes. Ei was cytogenetically studied on
three separate occasions and consistently contained both
male and female karyotypes in varying proportions(Fig.1).
Electron microscopy of these cell lines revealed many type
C virus particles in the extracellular space(Fig.2). The
cells from each cell line were 100% ATLA-positive when reacted by indirect immunofluorescence (Hinuma et al 1981)
with sera from ATL patients (Fig.3) but not with negative
control sera. These characterisitcs are shown in Table 1.

The present experiment was designed on the basis of our
previous findings that ATLV can be induced with phytohemag-
glutinin in short-term lymphocyte cultures from anti-ATLA
positive healthy persons (Miyoshi et al 1982a; Miyoshi et al
1982b) and that ATLV has capacity to transform normal human
T-cells in vitro apparently by cell-to-cell infection
(Miyoshi et al 1981b; Miyoshi et al 1982c). It was reasoned
that ATLV which might be similarly induced by alloantigenic
stimulation during mixed lymphocyte culture between anti-
ATLA positive and negative donors would transform either
autologous or allogeneic T-cells or both. Indeed, hetero-
sexual co-cultivation of lymphocytes from three seropositive
and two seronegative healthy persons gave rise to the isolation of three ATLV-producing T-cell lines. Two of them were

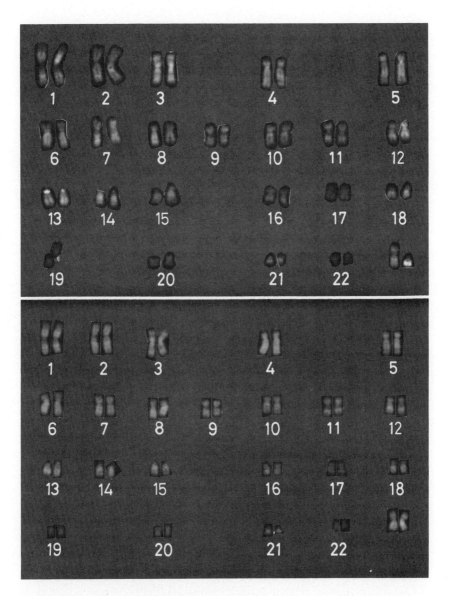

Fig. 1. Q-banded normal karyotypes of Ei showing a mixed population of male (uuper) and female (lower) cells.

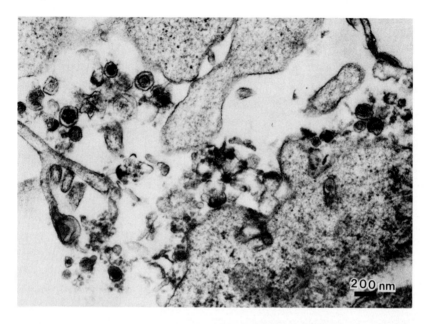

Fig. 2. Electron micrograph of Ei showing many type C virus particles in the extracellular space.

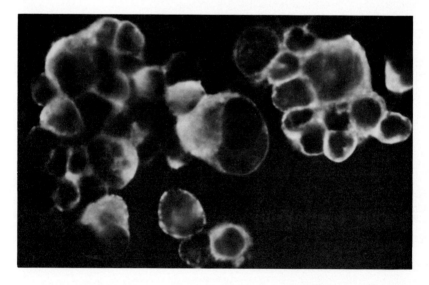

Fig. 3. Immunofluorescent micrograph of Ei showing ATLA in the cytoplasm of all cells.

Table I. ATLV-producing T-cell Lines Established by Mixed Lymphocyte Culture

Cell lines	Donors of mixed lymphocyte culture		Characteristics of cell lines[b]						
	Anti-ATLA positive females[a]	Anti-ATLA negative males	E[c]	Leu-1	OKI1	EBNA[d]	Karyotype	ATLV	ATLA
Ha	B	TK	86	80	88	Neg	46,XX	Pos	100
As	D	TK	85	90	91	Neg	46,XX	Pos	100
Ei	E	MF	52	84	100	Neg	46,XY/46,XX	Pos	100

a) For symbol identification, see reference Miyoshi et al 1982b.
b) Figures indicate percent of positive cells.
c) Spontaneous rosette formation with neuraminidase-treated sheep erythrocytes.
d) Epstein-Barr virus nuclear antigen.

derived from seropositive donors and the other consisted of
a mixed population of cells from seropositive and seronegative donors. These findings coincide with those of Gotoh et
al (1982) who obtained clonal cultures of ATLV-carrying T-
cells from anti-ATLA positive healthy adults. They reported
that the clones which were initiated and maintained with T-
cell growth factor (TCGF) became later TCGF-independent. In
contrast, no TCGF was used in our experiment. The mixed
lymphocyte culture method herein described provides a simple
means for the isolation of ATLV from anti-ATLA positive individuals.

The results reported in this paper extend our previous
observation that anti-ATLA positive healthy persons are
latent carriers of ATLV (Miyoshi et al 1982a; Miyoshi et al
1982b) and reemphasize the need for screening anti-ATLA pos-
tive blood donors (Saxinger, Gallo 1982). Transfusion of
ATLV-genome carrying lymphocytes into seronegative recipients would evoke an reaction in vivo similar to mixed lymphocyte culture and result in the infectious transmission of
ATLV from the donors to the recipients. This is consistent
with the data of Okochi (1982) that anti-ATLA seroconversion
occurred in three of six patients following blood transfusion from anti-ATLA positive donors.

The authors thank Drs. Masatoshi Fujishita, Shizuo
Yoshimoto, Ichiro Kubonishi and Takao Kitagawa for collaboration. This work was supported by Grants-in-Aid for Cancer
Research from the Japanese Ministry of Education, Science
and Culture, the Japanese Foundation for Multi-disciplinary
Treatment of Cancer and the Takamatsu Princess Cancer research Foundation.

Akagi T, Ohtsuki Y, Takahashi K, Kubonishi I, Miyoshi I (in
    press). Detection of type C virus particles in short-term
    cultured adult T-cell leukemia (ATL) cells. Lab Invest
Gotoh Y, Sugamura K, Hinuma Y (in press). Healthy carriers
    of a human retrovirus, adult T-cell leukemia virus (ATLV):
    Demonstration by clonal culture of ATLV-carrying T-cells
    from peripheral blood. Proc Natl Acad Sci USA
Hinuma Y, Gotoh Y, Sugamura K, Nagata K, Goto T, Nakai M,
    Kamada N, Matsumoto T, Kinoshita K (1982). A retrovirus
    associated with human adult T-cell leukemia: In vitro
    activation. Gann 73:341.

Hinuma Y, Nagata K, Hanaoka M, Nakai M, Matsumoto T, Kinoshita K, Shirakawa S, Miyoshi I (1981). Adult T-cell leukemia: Antigen in an ATL cell line and detection of antibodies to the antigen in human sera. Proc Natl Acad Sci USA 78:6476.

Miyoshi I, Fujishita M, Taguchi H, Ohtsuki Y, Akagi T, Morimoto YM, Nagasaki A (1982a). Caution against blood transfusion from donors seropositive to adult T-cell leukaemia-associated antigens. Lancet i:683.

Miyoshi I, Kubonishi I, Yoshimoto S, Akagi T, Ohtsuki Y, Shiraishi Y, Nagata K, Hinuma Y (1981a). Type C virus particles in a cord T-cell line derived by co-cultivating normal human cord leukocytes and human leukaemic T cells. Nature (London) 294:770.

Miyoshi I, Taguchi H, Fujishita M, Niiya K, Kitagawa T, Ohtsuki Y, Akagi T (1982b). Asymptomatic type C virus carriers in the family of an adult T-cell leukemia patient. Gann 73:339.

Miyoshi I, Taguchi H, Kubonishi I, Yoshimoto S, Ohtsuki Y, Akagi T, Shiraishi Y (1982c). Transformation of normal human lymphocytes by co-cultivation with a type C virus-producing human T-cell line. Proc Am Assoc Cancer Res 23:24

Miyoshi I, Yoshimoto S, Kubonishi I, Taguchi H, Shiraishi Y, Ohtsuki Y, Akagi T (1981b). Transformation of normal human cord lymphocytes by co-cultivation with a lethally irradiated human T-cell line carrying type C virus particles. Gann 72:997.

Okochi K (1982). Personal communication.

Poiesz BJ, Ruscetti FW, Gazdar AF, Bunn PA, Minna JD, Gallo RC (1980). Detection and isolation of type C retrovirus particles from fresh and cultured lymphocytes of a patient with cutaneous T-cell lymphoma. Proc Natl Acad Sci USA 77:7415.

Poiesz BJ, Ruscetti FW, Peitz MS, Kalyanaraman VS, Gallo RC (1981). Isolation of new type C retrovirus (HTLV) in primary uncultured cells of a patient with Sezary T-cell leukaemia. Nature (London) 294:268.

Sexinger WC, Gallo RC (1982). Possible risk to repients of blood from donors carrying serum markers of human T-cell leukaemia virus. Lancet i:1074.

ROUNDTABLE DISCUSSION

Oncogenes and Retroviruses: Evaluation of Basic Findings
and Clinical Potential, pages 253–272

ROUNDTABLE DISCUSSION

Dr. Frank J. Rauscher, Chairman

Participants: Dr. Alexander Bloch, Dr. Dani Paul
Bolognesi, Dr. John J. Burns, Dr. Myron Essex, Dr. Peter
J. Fischinger, Dr. George J. Galasso, Dr. Robert Gallo,
Dr. Jordan U. Gutterman, Dr. William S. Hayward, Dr.
Maurice R. Hilleman, Dr. Henry S. Kaplan, Dr. Werner H.
Kirsten, Dr. Arthur D. Levinson, Dr. Enrico Mihich, Dr.
Arnold I. Mittelman, Dr. Isao Miyoshi, Dr. Timothy E.
O'Connor, Dr. Howard Ozer, Dr. Harvey D. Preisler, Dr.
Ruth Sager, Dr. Thomas B. Shows

    I trust that this is going to be a quite informal
discussion that will provide each of the discussants an
opportunity to comment on anything that they have heard in
the last day and a half, or for that matter, to present
anything new and pertinent to the topic of our Symposium.
As Chairman, I would specifically request that we
emphasize the second part of what our program demands;
that is, the evaluation of basic findings that have been
presented in the light of their clinical potential. So
far we have had presentations of many elegant basic
findings but as yet relatively little discussion on what
this means for "people benefit". So I hope that we will
address the people benefit that will result from the
technologies and findings with oncogenes. Are there now
new strategies for cancer detection and prevention? Over
the past few days a number of us have had discussions of
the possibility of considering a vaccine against the HTLV
viruses that have been discussed here by Dr. Gallo and Dr.
Miyoshi. It would appear that this is not a realistic
option at this time in view of the relative incidence of
the disease. On the other hand, it is something that we
can begin to think about now that we would not even be
worthy of thought a few years ago. Is it realistic, for
instance, to believe that as we learn more about oncogenes
and their control in the genome, that we will be able to

apply that information to the prevention of cancer while learning how to control the switching mechanisms? I'd like some comment on that. Finally, what new strategies are there, if any, for treatment? Surely Dr. Kaplan and Dr. Mihich, among others, will wish to comment on that.

I think the panel, too, should consider input from the audience on these particular topics. Perhaps a good place to begin would be by reopening the discussion of Dr. Miyoshi's excellent paper and also the paper presented by Dr. Gallo.

Dr. Kaplan. My question is addressed to both Dr. Gallo and Dr. Miyoshi. Now that cloned full length DNA probes exist has the extent of homology between the HTLV isolates and the ATLV of Japan been examined and are they indeed identical? Can one now say with confidence that HTLV and ATLV essentially belong in the same family of viruses?

Dr. Rauscher. Dr. Gallo, would you care to first comment?

Dr. Gallo. Actually the data that is responsive to your question is addressed in a joint paper including Dr. Miyoshi and myself. The information that we presently have based on cloned probes or utilization of the monoclonal antibodies to the viral antigens indicate that each of the viruses from either this country or Japan are essentially identical and are also similar to the virus isolates we have been seeing in the Caribbean. They belong to a common family. Of course, we cannot yet say that at the nucleotide level they are identical, only at the detectable homology level. We can say that the virus isolates are as closely related as different isolates of the bovine leukemia virus and certainly more related than are the usual feline leukemia virus isolates as a group. However, as I stressed in my talk, exceptions have been seen. I mentioned an isolate from an individual in Israel with a retroperitoneal lymphoma of T-cells who had never left Israel, and also another individual with a benign T-cell leukemia from Seattle, Washington. These virus isolates are related but, nevertheless, are substantially different from the original HTLV isolates. Nevertheless, a substantial reaction between the proteins of these viruses and the original isolates has been found. These,

however, are exceptions. The original isolates from my
laboratory and those from the Japanese workers as tested
by cloned probes or with monoclonal antibodies appear to
be very closely related, if not identical.

Dr. Kirsten. I have another question for both Dr.
Gallo and Dr. Miyoshi. You both have mentioned that the
viruses are perhaps similar, possibly related to bovine
leukemia virus or leukosis virus. As you are aware, in
the bovine leukosis, as it occurs in nature, there is as
yet an unidentified serum factor which somehow interferes
with virus production and therefore for virus production
one has to place the cells in culture where the putative
serum factor is diluted. Question: Is there a similar
phenomenon observed that you could tell us about with
relation to these adult T-cell leukemias? I should also
mention that this serum factor exists in mice as has been
described by Dr. Bolognesi.

Dr. Gallo. I should also mention that Dr. Fischinger
at an earlier date has described an inhibitory factor for
virus production. First, let me deal with the
relationship of HTLV to bovine leukemia virus. I think I
have got myself into trouble in the past by constantly
referring to similarities of the biology of this virus,
HTLV, and the biology of bovine leukosis. Saying this
frequently enough has caused some reviewers to state that
the virus we are dealing with is, in fact, bovine leukemia
virus. That patently is absurd. No significant close
relationships exist between HTLV and bovine leukosis virus
except by amino acid sequencing of some of the gag genes.
There is a distant homology between the viruses in the
amino acid sequencing of P24, particularly at the carboxy
terminus of the gag gene. Steve Oroszelan has almost
completed sequencing of the P15 protein and, not
surprisingly, relationships were found since that protein
is conserved among most mammalian retroviruses. Except
for this homology, little other relationships can be found
but the biology, however, of both viruses is quite
reminescent. Now, specifically dealing with your question
of inhibitors. I would prefer to delay the answer, but a
preliminary answer is yes, there is an inhibitory factor
present which prevents expression of HTLV. We have
detected such a factor but we have not yet chemically
defined it since we are in the midst of purifying it. I
can say it is not an immunoglobulin or an interferon but

it inhibits expression of the virus in the primary fresh tumor. One can take the primary fresh tumor, place it in media in the absence of calf serum and see the expression of retrovirus particles, sometimes even without the induction of growth by TCGF. So, contrary to what I felt in the past, it is simply not a matter of getting the cells to grow with TCGF. Part of the mechanism for virus expression requires removing the inhibitor. Our studies fully accord with the earlier precedent from the studies of Dr. Fischinger and Dr. Bolognesi in the mouse, and also in the cow. However, Dr. Kirsten, I believe you know more about the cow factor since you recently visited with investigators working in bovine leukosis, so I really haven't much new on it.

Dr. Fischinger. I would like to address a different topic. I think it is quite remarkable that with the HTLV one gets almost instant immortalization of these cells on infection and when they are examined they very much resemble the leukemic cell population. In comparison with animal models, it would be very interesting to see whether or not during the phase of initial benign lymphocytosis the integration of the genome occurs in the polyclonal state or whether, as the disease develops, there is a monoclonal type of integration in specific site. I would like to specifically address this question to the tissue culture model and ask, as one develops lines after the initial co-cultivations, are these monoclonal in terms of site integration.

Dr. Gallo. With respect to the experiments in cord blood the cells initially transformed by HTLV are initially polyclonal but the final cell line ends up monoclonal after co-cultivation. With regard to tumors that we see in vivo, they have all been monoclonal, and that has also been the experience of the Japanese workers. We have not until recently been in a position to identify anyone who is in an early phase but one of our patients that I have briefly alluded to may be in a pre-leukemic stage by the criteria I gave, and we are currently examing the integration sites in these patients' T-lymphocytes. We will have to await the outcome of these studies to see whether the cells of these individuals are in fact polyclonal.

Dr. Bolognesi. I would like to address a question to Dr. Essex. Since he has been studying the expression of viral antigens, I will particularly welcome his comments on the issue of what kind of expression by HTLV either of its structural components or induced components could provide strategies for any kind of immunotherapy considerations in man. Would you make a few comments of what possible targets for immunotherapy may current exist.

Dr. Essex. We do find that there are some species of proteins in labelled HTLV as shed from metabolically labelled human tumor cells that are regularly detected by antibodies from either patient sera or sera from people that have been exposed to the virus. Some of these particular protein antigens are expressed on the surface of the cultured tumor cells. An important question then is, to what extent are they expressed on the fresh tissue of the tumors and whether they might be targets for future immunodiagnosis. The fascinating point of the HTLV system is the apparent monoclonality of the tumor that is associated apparently with a very long latent period for the disease. This reminds me of the very exciting studies of Dr. Hayward and his group of the B-cell lymphomas in the chicken which involve promoter insertion of the virus adjacent to the myc gene resulting in expression of myc RNA. I emphasize this because as far as I know most naturally occurring human cancers are monoclonal tumors, not polyclonal tumors of the type that are seen with rapidly transforming viruses in cell culture. The HTLV tumors like the bovine, feline and avian B-cell lymphomas all have long latent periods prior to development and result as monoclonal tumors. I am excited by Dr. Hayward's results where in some infections with V-myc after relatively brief latent periods there are examples of the development of tumors associated with expression of myc RNA and that these tumors are in fact monoclonal. If I am correct in this and the latent period is indeed short, we would have to postulate that there are preferential integration sites. That assumption, however, critically depends on how long the latent period for the tumor is and whether the kinetics of cell growth would allow one to visualize the development of one altered cell to the point where you could call it a tumor in the time frame. I deem this an important issue and I would like appealing to the other discussants as to its importance. I would like however, to also raise the issue that the myc gene may not be one that is detected by transfection assays and that this discrepancy poses a dilemma in our evaluation of human tumor materials. I would like Dr. Hayward's comments on the latent period of the V-myc initiated B-cell lymphomas.

Dr. Hayward. I would like to emphasize that the results to which you referred are somewhat preliminary. Our indications are that some of the tumors induced by MC29 are clonal. As yet we have no evidence at all that there is a specific integration site. The clonality of these tumors could be explained by a number of possible sequence of events. For example, if expression of myc alone is not sufficient to induce frank tumors, it may be that there is a selection among the population of cells infected with MC29 for a second event. This would be analogous to what Cooper has described in the lymphomas induced by ALV. Thus, among the expanded population one or a few cells would undergo a second change. All that clonality really means is that whatever leads to transformation is perhaps a rare enough event that the final tumor is the result of a single infection and that perhaps the transformation itself is not rapidly spread by recruiting neighboring cells. One could explain the phenomenon simply by an initial infection and an inefficient spread of MC29 virus to neighboring cells simply because there is not a helper virus present. MC29 of course is a defective virus that requires a helper. The latency period of MC29 induced lymphomas is of the order of one to two months in our experiments. Now this of course is somewhat longer than that seen with Rous sarcoma virus where essentially no latency period exists and tumors are detected within days or even a week after infection with RSV. Is there any other aspect of this that you think I should address?

Dr. Essex. I assume that one of the steps that will be addressed by many people in the future is the expression of proteins related to some of the onc genes. Clearly the detection of proteins expressed by the myc gene is very important since this is one of the genes regularly expressed in a lot of human lymphoid cells. Are there approaches that you are aware of using synthetic antigen technology or antisera directed to regions of the myc specific sequence that you think will be used in the future to detect proteins associated with the myc gene?

Dr. Hayward. Are you asking whether there is an antibody against myc and whether I can envision an approach based on this antibody?

Dr. Essex. Yes.

Dr. Hayward. I am not aware of an antibody against myc. We are trying to raise antibodies in common with about 10 other laboratories. Clearly, somebody soon should have an effective antibody against the myc protein.

Dr. Levinson. I would like to comment on this topic. Our approach to identify these oncogenic products has been to express the products of the gene in E. coli and then to purify the product. In collaborative studies with Dr. Bishop we have raised antibodies against the polypeptides produced in E. coli and have identified products coded for by the erb locus in chicken and also the myb. So far our attempts to express myc in E. coli have not been successful. It it not clear why, but it may well be that myc is not tolerated well in E. coli.

Dr. Rauscher. Dr. Miyoshi, I found your paper very interesting. Permit me a question. Is the Japanese Macaque the only subhuman primate that you have tested so far that you have found to be positive? Are you aware of other studies of this type in either Japan or this country testing primates?

Dr. Miyoshi. No. So far we have tested only the serum Rhesus of a few. These were negative.

Dr. Sager. What impressed me in the data on the HTLV was the large number of carriers and the fact that when this virus is present antibodies can be produced and there is frequently no disease. This is reminescent of the SV40 situation in which the same is true and highlights the fact that human cells carry some kind of suppressor mechanism which protects us and explains why, in fact, we are able to gather here today. I would like to raise the point that an approach which have been comparatively neglected and which I would really like to emphasize for everyone's attention is the possibility cells carry a suppressor gene or genes. If these genes can be identified, this would provide a new kind of therapeutic approach. I would like to ask regarding the pedigrees of the families in which the HTLV virus has been found. An analysis of these pedigrees might reveal that people who get the disease have actually segregated out the suppressor gene.

Dr. Raushcer. That's a very interesting point. Dr. Gallo and Dr. Miyoshi, have you in fact enough data on the pedigrees of the families to address this question?

Dr. Gallo. I would like to make a statement that would put this in perspective. In our group we have never seen a Caucasian with the HTLV virus who does not have disease.

Dr. Rauscher. Repeat that.

Dr. Gallo. We have as yet seen nobody who is white, who has the virus, who does not have leukemia or lymphoma.

Dr. Rauscher. That is extremely interesting.

Dr. Gallo. I don't want to make too much at this point, for I suspect that HTLV has relatively recently been introduced in some places in the world. That's our data to date. The virus is endemic in certain regions. In an endemic region such as Venezuela where the virus is detected in the normal population, it's in the Black population. Now, obviously, some Caucasians must have antibodies to the virus. We simply have not as yet looked widely enough. We do not know enough yet to speak of cancer markers and genetic markers. As yet we have not found a susceptibility factor. It may be noted that the level of virus infection observed in the Japanese population results in leukemia, is rather comparable to that seen in production of overt bovine leukosis on infection with bovine leukemia virus. I mention this because there is evidence that genetic factors in some herds of cows produce resistance to bovine leukosis.

Dr. Ozer. I would like to ask Drs. Miyoshi and Gallo whether they have any data available on the relation of gamma interferon system and HTLV. Does HTLV effect gamma interferon production? Are there different levels in the patients who have it versus those family members who have antibody?

Dr. Miyoshi. We have no data on the production of gamma interferon from our cell lines. To date we have tested only whether fibroblast interferon inhibits the production of the type C particles from our cells. In fact the continued presence of fibroblast interferon does inhibit production of the type C particles. Interestingly, in the presence of interferon the virus particles were internalized within the cytoplasm and not the extracellular space. There was very strong production of viral antigen despite presence of interferon.

Dr. Rauscher. Thank you, Dr. Miyoshi. Dr. Gallo, have you further information relating to interferon?

Dr. Gallo. Yes. The experience in our laboratory has been similar. Presence of interferon blocks translation of a lot of viral messages and you get accumulation of incomplete virus particles. Regarding production of gamma interferon, it should be borne in mind that tumor cells are activated T-cells. One would expect them to produce gamma interferon. The answer is that sometimes one does find gamma interferon made by the cells and sometimes one does not. We have as yet to perform really sophisticated studies that would make a clear correlation with the role of the virus in interferon production.

Dr. Shows. I'd like to make a few comments on suppressors, carriers, and genetic markers that the last few speakers have mentioned. There is currently a poverty of genetic markers based on the usual marker system of enzymes and surface antigens. Now, however, we have the possibility of examining DNA polymorphisms which have been alluded to only once in this meeting. Now there are available polymorphisms that are detectable in DNA fractions obtained by restriction enzymes. These polymorphisms involve nucleotide substitutions or rearrangements. If one looks at the emerging data from polymorphism studies, one sees that in at least every thousand nucleotide base sequence, a base change can be detected among the natural population. It is important to note that we can now follow any given family by individual polymorphisms. Let me now turn to the topic brought up by Dr. Sager. Clearly, there are human chromosomes that contain genes that suppress tumors. Her suggestion that these suppressors can operate on oncogenes may well be possible. It's a good bet. She mentioned data involving

chromosome 11. There are, however, additional chromosomes
that have suppressors. Klinger, in collaboration with
members of our laboratory, used cell hybrids that have
been injected into nude mice and these studies have
detected suppressors on chromosomes 11, 2, 9, 10 and 17.
Let me remind you that in this Conference we have heard
from Dr. Sakaguchi and his coworkers that sarc is on
chromosome 20 and Kirsten ras is on chromosome 12 and that
myc is on chromosome 8.

Dr. Mihich. As a result of this Symposium, it seems
reasonable to conclude that progress has been made towards
the recognition of the uncertainties and yet exciting
potentialities of this area of molecular biology in terms
of possible future therapeutic exploitation. It seems to
me that three major, perhaps naive, sets of questions need
to be answered, namely: 1) Because of the unique need for
3T3 cells as target of transformation, is the role of
oncgene an "artifact" or is the system actually
representing an exquisite counterpart of the rare human
cell that can indeed undergo carcinogenic transformation?
I like to believe the latter, and also that other target
cells will be found which are transformed by genetic
material other than that identified to date. Yet this set
of questions needs to be answered. 2) In those cases
where the overactivity of oncgenes is regulated by a unit
like the LTR, is this regulation required to maintain the
neoplastic state or not? It is apparent that oncgene
hyperactivity is required, but as these genes do not seem
to be different (or too different) from counterparts
present in normal tissues, they may again provide
essentially quantitative differences for therapeutic
exploitation. The recent observation by Weinberg's group
that the "has" gene present in bladder tumor cells differs
from its normal counterpart by expressing valine instead
of glycine is promising. Should the role of this
difference be understood and should other such differences
be found in other systems, it may be possible to identify
exploitable specificities at the level of oncgenes too.
3) Of the numerous oncgenes products being identified
which ones are critical for the maintenance of the
neoplastic state and thus may provide sites for
therapeutic intervention?

The answer to these questions may provide important
clues towards ultimate therapeutic exploitation based on a

modification of oncgene regulation and function.

Dr. Preisler. I would like to suggest the utility of human chronic myeloid leukemia as an excellent model for the study of the expression of onc genes in neoplasia. First I would note that the disease is a two-step process. In the first step, the chronic phase, one has abnormal regulation of proliferation but the cells that are examined appear to be normally differentiated. In the second event, which involves every single patient, there is a loss of the ability to differentiate and it is this second characteristic that ultimately leads to death. The chromosomes involved are very well characterized. Chromosome 22 is involved in every single case of chronic myelocytic leukemia. Chromosome 17, or a trisomy of chromosome 8, all of which have been mentioned during the last two days as being the sites of oncogenes or the potential sites of suppressor genes, are involved in the blast crisis. Since this type of cellular evolution occurs in each case, it provides a population which is well suited for the studies on expression of onc genes. I would like to ask Dr. Gallo to comment on this in view of his experience with transfection of the HL60. And I would also like to suggest to Dr. Aaronson that one of the reasons for not picking up transfection of the myc gene in the chronic stages is that perhaps a more appropriate time for examination of cells would be in the blast crisis when two Philadelphia chromosomes are present. Maybe the gene dosage phenomenon is involved.

Dr. Gallo. As yet we have no information on the protein product of the transfecting entity in transfection experiments. Dr. Weinberg's experiments on transfection with HL60 suggest that the myc is amplified, that it is a homolog of a retroviral onc, and that it is expressed in moderate amounts and that it can be turned off by inducing differentiation of the normal phenotype of these cells. All these findings suggest that the myc gene is likely to be important. I would agree with Dr. Preisler that CML as a disease entity has tended to be forgotten. With regard to chromosome 22, the sis onc is present on this chromosome. Sis and its products are currently under intense investigation. The sis sequences have been completely sequenced in Dr. Aaronson's lab and also in our laboratory. Antibodies to the sis proteins are being made in Dr. Aaronson's lab and Dr. Oroszlan is making antibodies to these products at Frederick. The findings to date suggest that there is no expression of sis in CML chronic or blast phases. Preliminary information from other laboratories suggest that expression of an onc may be influenced by chromosomal translocations.

Dr. Mittelman. Let me turn to the presentation of Dr. Garth Anderson as a potential model for the topics that we are discussing. I believe that the LDH_k described by Dr. Garth Anderson may provide a unique marker for a variety of neoplasias in man. The implications, I believe, are really quite profound both theoretically and practically. From a practical point of view, one can readily see how one can assay and correlate LDH_k with disease states. On the theoretical level, I believe a more fascinating question is, is this a new version of the older speculations of Otto Warburg? Have we finally seen what this particular enzyme, LDH_k, an achilles heel in the spectrum of neoplastic diseases?

Dr. Bloch. Following up this line, I would like to raise a question which I know is also shared by Dr. Mihich on the possible role that oncogenes play as targets for selective chemotherapeutic intervention. As Dr. Gallo has already emphasized, the normal cell is distinguished from that of the tumor cell by the fact that it does not switch off in G1 to go from proliferation to differentiation. In contrast the normal cell replicates for a few cycles and then differentiates to a mature stage which is accompanied by cessation of proliferation. Now, various factors, such as colony stimulating factor, signal the direction at which this event occurs. The oncogenes apparently play a role in holding the cells at a particular stage. Differentiation inducers, in contrast, move the cell forward. The question which I would raise is whether the cell has lost the ability to respond to these proliferation signals. I would point to the ML1, a myeloblastic leukemia cell line, which is arrested at a stage earlier than is Dr. Gallo's HL60 (which is promyelocytic human leukemia line). When these ML1 cells are stimulated with mitogen-conditioned medium they readily differentiate to clear cut components of the monocyte-phagocyte complex. Within a day complete differentiation of these cells to completely mature cells occurs. These final cells are, of course, terminally differentiated. What these findings imply is that the

response to the exogenous stimulus is still retained and
that what is needed is an increased complement of stimulus
in order to bring about the differentiations. One could
express this by saying that there is a certain amount of
insensitivity of the tumor cell to established levels of
the stimuli. As Dr. Gallo has implied with respect to
findings on HL60 in his laboratory, and as Dr. Friend
showed many years ago, such cells can respond very readily
to the clinically effective antitumor agents with rapid
induction of differentiation. An interesting recent
finding in our laboratory is that it is that only agents
that interfere with DNA synthesis, not those that
interfere with protein or RNA synthesis, that are capable
of producing this induction. This suggests that
interference with DNA synthesis inhibits the formation of
the onc gene product. Keeping this in mind, both drugs as
well as natural factors allow the retransformation of the
malignant cell to the normal cell type. We can visualize
the handle at chemotherapeutic intervention.

Dr. Rauscher. Thank you Dr. Bloch. I think Dr.
Galasso has a comment.

Dr. Galasso. In an earlier discussion Dr. Mihich
referred to himself as a pro-neophyte in this field.
Consequently, I must regard myself as a pre-proneophyte.
But perhaps it is useful to have people like Dr. Mihich
and myself at meetings. Perhaps we still don't understand
the trees, not to mind the forest, but I have been very
interested and excited by the results presented here. I
would like to address Dr. Rauscher's question regarding
"people benefits", particularly in the context of the
recent findings by Dr. Gallo and Dr. Miyoshi. One of the
things that I see that should be done almost immediately
is to try to develop a quick and easy type of assay for
the agent so that bloods of blood donors can be examined.
I visualize that as we now screen blood for hepatitis B
antigen we should soon be testing for agents such as the
HTLV. The clustering of the virus and the facile in vitro
transformation of cells lead one to believe that this will
be very important thing and we should be looking at
examination for HTLV in blood banks. This is an important
first step in direct people benefit. The next step is
clearly further sera epidemiology relating to HTLV. The
present data on endemic areas and familial relationships
are intriguing. If, in fact, people who have antibody do

eventually develop disease, we need not only longitudinal but horizontal and longitudinal epidemiology. This will be important later in evaluation of potential approaches to vaccines. I would also like to pick up on the point made in Dr. Gallo's talk on the use of probes. As we develop better probes we may well be finding more and more viruses in tumors than the ones that have been mentioned to date.

Dr. Kaplan. A brief comment on the question that was just raised. A recent report from Japan describes a blood bank of sera that had been stored for possible hepatitis B carriers. With this population they identified a group of sera that were positive for HTLA antigen. At the time of the paper two patients were identified – and other patients have been found – who actually developed the T-cell lymphoma. So we already have in hand a model for the question raised by Dr. Galasso.

Dr. Preisler. What happened to the people who received blood from these donors?

Dr. Kaplan. I think Dr. Miyoshi's report on that may have more data. There are indications that formed blood elements in transfusion may transmit the virus.

Dr. Miyoshi. In our two cases I followed one the patients for six months. This patient has been under treatment for dialysis for renal trouble but during this period we did not demonstrate cell conversion. We also did not detect positively the antibody in this patient. In the second patient the receipient was already antibody positive so we cannot determine the effect of the blood transfusion. In other studies in Japan as a follow-up of positive blood transfusions 3 out of 6 people who received positive blood showed positive antibody production.

Dr. Rauscher. Dr. John Burns, from the viewpoint of the pharmaceutical industry, have you got any thoughts on this or other matters?

Dr. Burns. I would compare what I have heard over the past few days to almost a generalized field theory of cancer. A lot of things are beginning to fall in place, obviously, a lot of answers are still awaited. The field of onc genes represents an excellent example where basic research from a number of different areas coincides with the development of new technology to result in a new synthesis. As of today I would be a little hesitant in marking out road for future development of onc genes for human betterment. Some of the things that have come into my mind over the past few days have been the effects of retinoids on differentiation. Is there something in all of this that could tell us more about explaining some of the role of various factors   I would also like to mention the potential effects of Vitamin D_3 on metabolites on differentiation or proliferation. I think that we see here is a gathering of information that may lead to new syntheses. Ultimately, this will lead to new strategies.

Dr. Rauscher. Thank you, Dr. Burns. Dr. Gutterman, I would welcome your perspective.

Dr. Gutterman. As a clinical scientist who has been involved with research on biological approaches to the control of tumor growth with agents such as the interferons, this meeting has been extraordinarily exciting. There is little doubt in my mind that we are on the brink of important diagnostic and possibly therapeutic advances in clinical oncology based on the emerging knowledge of oncogenes, tumor viruses and transforming growth factors. As one who has had experience in bringing new biotechnology from the laboratory into the clinic, I think that a close interrelationship between academic and industrial research laboratories, industry and clinical research programs is essential to move the oncogene field quickly to the bedside for the benefit of present and future cancer patients.

The study of oncogenes and their products will have applicability in the clinic first as potential diagnostic tools. I was impressed that only a small number of oncogenes identified with currently identified retroviral probes may be involved with human malignancy. For example, the ras system may turn out to be quite important in human epithelial malignancies. The myc system seems important in hematological disorders. Close collaboration between clinical oncologists, retrovirologists and molecular biologists should begin to categorize fresh human tumors using monoclonal antibodies against identified oncogene proteins in Western blot analysis. Characterization of oncogene expression by the study of

RNA from fresh tumor cells by Northern blot analysis as
reported at this meeting, should be expanded.

I feel that we might come up with a new classification
of tumors based on the expression of oncogene products.
This may be of particular therapeutic importance because
of the possibility of interfering with specific
biochemical and enzymatic pathways, depending upon which
oncogene product is expressed in a particular malignancy.

The point mutation reported at this meeting opens up
the possibility that specific inherited or acquired
molecular defects predisposing to a specific malignancy
may be identified by restriction enzyme analysis with
small amounts of cellular material.

What about therapy? Here I think the outlook is
futuristic but realistic and as exciting as the potential
diagnostic applications. I think we will be able to
develop more precise biochemical targets for therapy in
cancer. As we have heard, the promoter insertion
mechanism may be applicable to several forms of
hematologic tumors. Human solid tumors such as colon,
lung, and bladder cancers are probably rarely induced by
viruses but certainly it appears that specific oncogenes
recognized by retroviral probes are activated. We already
know a fair amount about the biochemistry of certain
oncogene products, the possibility of interfering with
tyrosine phosphorylation or other specific enzymatic
targets is intriguing. Thus, the biochemist may have new
and specific therapeutic targets to think about.

The Gallo paper illustrates the interrelationships of
a human retrovirus infection, tumor growth, and the
production of growth factors. The possibility of
interfering with growth factors or transforming substances
by developing receptor antagonists is intriguing. Thus,
instead of interfering with DNA synthesis, the target of
most chemotherapeutic agents, we should be thinking about
specific enzymatic or receptor targets.

I feel we already may be interfering with oncogene
expression with agents such as the interferons. I have
been intrigued by our own clinical studies carried out by
Dr. Quesada and me, in which malignant lymphomas and renal
tumors appear to be two of the most sensitive malignancies

to human leukocyte interferon. I have asked myself what common denominator could there be between renal tumors, which are normally resistant to all forms of systemic therapy, and human lymphomas? Lymphomas and renal tumors are often caused by chronic RNA tumor viruses in avian systems. Could it be that leukocyte interferon has specificity for the same oncogene product which may be commonly activated in these two tumors? There is emerging evidence that leukocyte interferon may interfere with the protein kinase activity of pp60^{src}. This observation goes along with the knowledge that interferon strengthens the cytoskeleton of transformed cells.

As George Klein has pointed out, many malignant disorders in man may be related to the expression of oncogenes and their proteins at an abnormal time in the cell cycle. Such events could be occurring in chronic myelogenous leukemia in which the translocation of parts of chromosome 22 to chromosome 9 appears in most cases (Philadelphia chromosome). In the chronic hyperproliferative phase, this disorder is primarily characterized by excess proliferation of myeloid tissue. Eventually the disease progresses to a more malignant acute variety known as blastic crisis. Thus, there may be genes in chromosome 22, chromosome 9 or both that are involved with myeloid proliferation and differentiation. My colleague Dr. Talpaz and I have been treating patients with chronic myelogeneous leukemia with leukocyte interferon and have achieved complete hematologic control in most patients thus far. It appears that we have been able to "reset the thermostat" and achieve a more normal regulation of myeloid proliferation. We may modify the expression of an oncogene by a natural regulatory molecule such as interferon. The abl gene is apparently located at the translocation site on chromosome 9. It is interesting that the genes for production of leukocyte and fibroblast interferons are present on the short arm of chromosome 9. The translocation of 22 usually occurs at the end of the long arm of chromosome 9. Whether this translocation can disrupt the regulation of genes on the short arm, I'm not sure. The Philadelphia chromosome defect can sometimes involve chromosomes other than 9.

Over the next few years, as the molecular events in the evolution of specific malignancies are elucidated, new and novel diagnostic and therapeutic approaches should lead to important advances in our quest for the control of human cancer.

Finally, I would like to make a comment about translocation of chromosomes interfering with the function of normal regulatory genes. Dr. Talpaz and I have treated several patients with chronic myelogenous leukemia with Philadelphia chromosome + (22:9 translocation). In most instances we have been able to reregulate the phenotypic manifestations of chronic myelogenous leukemia which is manifested by excess proliferation and a partial block in differentiation of myeloid elements. Could it be that the 22:9 translocation has disrupted the role of leukocyte interferons in the control of myeloid proliferation? Recent evidence has shown that the genes for leukocyte interferon production are located on chromosome 9. I think we may even be able to use onc gene products as therapy if their presence has been blocked and their expression is important for differentiation and arrest of proliferation.

Dr. Rauscher. Thank you, Dr. Gutterman. Dr. Kaplan, are there any closing remarks you would like to share with us?

Dr. Kaplan. Well, Dr. Rauscher, being an iconoclast, I may make two remarks that may well be inappropriate. Like the little boy who wrote a book review on crocodiles in which he stated that the book had taught him more about crocodiles than he had wanted to know, I would have to say that I have learned more about genes that further transform the already partially transformed NIH3T3 cell than I really wanted to know. My second comment is that careful analysis suggests that although tremendous emphasis has been placed on genes, I think Dr. Ruth Sager was right on the mark when she emphasized that it is not the genes per say but rather a disturbance of the gene or a switching of some kind having to do with regulation of expression of genes that is important. Now, this is a very welcome remark on the one hand but on the other, it's rather deflating because even when I went to medical school - which is many more years than I care to remember - I was taught that cancer is a disturbance of the regulation of the growth of the cell and therefore in a sense we have come full circle with our new-found knowledge.

Dr. Rauscher. Thank you, Dr. Kaplan. Dr. O'Connor, before I call upon you to make the last comments, which is appropriate, I do want to thank you and Dr. Gerald Murphy, Director of RPMI, on behalf of the audience and all of us here for having arranged this Conference and for your hospitality. Would you care to share some comments with us?

Dr. O'Connor. This meeting was addressed to an overview on oncogenes and retroviruses. We have heard a great deal about oncogenes and the first well-authenticated isolation of a retrovirus associated with human neoplasia. Now all of this is very important. Yet to me one of the fascinating aspects of the meeting was that a subcomponent of the integrated retroviral DNA, the long terminal repeat (LTR) segment, finally came into prominence in this meeting. We have heard some fascinating data of how particular regions of the LTR have a functional role in regulation. I am reflecting among the many excellent papers on that of Dr. Ann Skalka, where she presented data showing the sequences upstream from the promoter region as having a role almost as important as the onc gene itself in cellular transformation.

I should also mention that perhaps one of the areas that we did not go into in sufficient depth in the meeting was the role of a particular type of retrovirus, the mammary tumor viruses, in neoplasia. Recently there have been some very interesting reports on the structure of the more complex LTRs of these mammary tumor viruses. These new findings could have a profound effect on our approaches to human mammary carcinoma. I have a suspicion that some of us will return to the laboratories from this meeting for a fresh look at some other areas than the ones dealt with at this meeting and reexamine these cancers in a fresh perspective.

Finally, I am intrigued by the role that surprise holds for all of us in cancer research. In view of the data on the expression of onc genes in neoplasia, I suspect that many of us would have expected a demonstration of a direct role for an onc gene in tumors associated with an authenticated human retrovirus isolate. Yet the tumor associated with HTLV appears to involve a terminally differentiated T-cell and may possibly arise from expression of inappropriate levels of

TCGF. Clearly we should be prepared for further surprises.

On behalf of my associates at RPMI, I wish to express my thanks to the participants and audience for joining us in this stimulating Workshop.

Index

PROGRESS IN CLINICAL AND BIOLOGICAL RESEARCH